Distinc

OSCES IN

SPECIALTIES

Smash Specialties.

Muhammad Najim *BSc (Hons)*

Riham Rabee *BSc (Hons)*

Faisal Al-Mayahi *BSc (Hons)*

David Zargaran *BSc (Hons)*

Muhammad Ashraf *BSc (Hons)*

Rula Najim *MBBS BSc AICSM MRCPUK DCCM*

Editors   Alexander Zargaran

Ibrahim Al-Mayahi

i

CONTENTS PAGE

CONTRIBUTORS

This book would not have reached its present high standard without the excellent contribution made by our mentors. We like to thank the following for their contributions, help and guidance:

Dr Zuhair Najim   *MBBS MRCPUK DPD DCD PGDD*

Dr Sam Chabuk   *MBBS BSc*

Dr Omar Taha   *MBBS BSc*

Dr. Mohammad Mahmud   *MBBS BSc MRCPUK*

Dr Rana Najim   *MBBS BSc (Hons)*

Dr Fatima Alm   *BDS MJDF RCS*

Maroof Ahmed   *BSc (Hons)*

Yusuf Sherwani   *BSc (Hons)*

Hamid Habib   *BSc*

Sarah Najim

Nuha Rabee

PREFACE

Distinction for OSCEs in Specialties was created with the vision of producing a handbook to guide medical students through the daunting prospect of OSCEs in Specialties. This book is intended for students studying for OSCEs and post-graduate PACES, comprehensively providing the knowledge required to achieve Distinctions across all specialty stations – Paediatrics, Obstetrics & Gynaecology, and Psychiatry. This book was written by Imperial College Teaching Fellows and medical students achieving Distinctions in their PACES examinations.

This is the first book to comprehensively address the following for all common presenting complaints in the three core specialties:

- Detailed history questions to be elicited including presenting complaint, history of presentation, past medical history, drug history & social history.
- Examination findings and guides to practical procedures.
- Investigations, including special tests.
- Management in line with the latest up-to-date NICE guidelines.
- Simplifies difficult conversations by providing counselling scripts.
- Memorable mnemonics are used throughout the book to aid memory retention.

The authors were faced with a problem that every medical student faces, in that no single resource contains all of the above in an organised and succinct manner. This simplifies revision and saves valuable time in collating everything you need to know for your OSCEs in one place. *Distinction for OSCEs in Specialties* prides itself in providing the following key features specific to each specialty:

Psychiatry:
- ICD-10 and DSM-5 criteria for establishing diagnosis.
- Biopyschosocial stratified approach taken towards management.

Obstetrics & Gynaecology:
- Latest RCOG 2015 guidelines used for investigation and management.

Paediatrics:
- Latest British Thoracic Society (BTS) and British Society for Paediatric Endocrinology and Diabetes (BSPED) Guidelines for paediatric emergencies such as Asthma and Diabetic Ketoacidosis.

Distinction for OSCEs in Specialties has been carefully designed to a concise length, realistically providing students with the ability to commit the book to memory and achieve top marks. We encourage students to read over *Distinction for OSCEs in Specialties* multiple times to consolidate their learning and to then apply their knowledge to clinical scenarios.

We hope this book will be as useful to you as it has been to us and to our many students. We wish you all the best on your road to clinical excellence!

FOREWORD

Distinction for OSCEs in Specialties has been written by clinicians, medical students and teaching fellows from Imperial College London who understand what medical schools like to assess. Therefore, this book serves as an up to date and universally applicable resource. As an examiner, I believe *Distinction for OSCEs in Specialties* has all the information required to achieve Distinctions and beyond.

There a large number of OSCE resources available for Medicine and Surgery, however this has not been the case for the Specialties until now. *Distinction in OSCEs for Specialties* fulfils a significant gap in literature for medical students and doctors. It helps bridge the gap between the textbooks and the OSCEs, providing a template with the key questions you need to ask for all the main presenting complaints in Obstetrics & Gynaecology, Paediatrics and Psychiatry.

The chapters bring together a wealth of knowledge from authoritative sources including NICE and the Royal Colleges. This allows students aiming for top marks to access the most up to date guideline-based investigations and management, making *Distinction for OSCEs in Specialties* applicable for both OSCEs and PACES examinations.

The success of *Distinction in OSCEs for Specialties* in enabling the authors to achieve Distinctions in their clinical examinations is why I hope this book is adopted in all medical schools across the country to assist every medical student in their journey to achieving Distinctions.

Dr Ban Al-Saffar, *MB ChB MRCPUK*
Consultant, Elderly Medicine Department
Queen Elizabeth Hospital London

Psychiatry

AD	Alzheimer's Disease
ADHD	Attention Deficit Hyperactivity Disorder (Hyperkinetic Syndrome)
ADL	Activities of Daily Living
AMTS	Abbreviated Mental Test Score
BDZ	Benzodiazepine
CAMHS	Child and Adolescent Mental Health Service
CBT	Cognitive Behavioural Therapy
CVA	Cerebrovascular Accident
DT	Delirium Tremens
DSM 5	Diagnostic and Statistical Manual of Mental Disorders, Fifth Edition
ECT	Electroconvulsive Therapy
GAD	Generalised Anxiety Disorder
ICD10	International Statistical Classification of Diseases and Related Health Problems
LT	Long-Term
OCD	Obsessive Compulsive Disorder
OD	Overdose
PDD	Parkinson's Disease Dementia
PTSD	Post-Traumatic Stress Disorder
SSRI	Selective Serotonin Reuptake Inhibitor
TCA	Tricyclic Antidepressant
VD	Vascular Dementia

Obstetrics & Gynaecology

ART	Anti-Retroviral Therapy
CTPA	Computed Tomography Pulmonary Angiography
BG	Blood Glucose

C/S	Caesarean Section
DVT	Deep vein thrombosis
GDM	Gestational Diabetes
HAART	Highly Active Anti-Retroviral Therapy
HELLP	Haemolysis Elevated Liver enzymes Low Platelet count
HSV	Herpes Simplex Virus
LMP	Last menstrual period
LMWH	Low Molecular Weight Heparin
RPOC	Retained Product of Conception
SFH	Symphysis Fundal Height
SGA	Small for Gestational Age
TED Stockings	Thromboembolic Deterrent Stockings
VD	Vaginal Delivery
V/Q Scan	Ventilation Perfusion Scan

Paediatrics

APLS	Antiphospholipid Syndrome
BR	Bilirubin
CVA	Cerebrovascular Accident
DAT	Direct Antiglobulin test
DKA	Diabetic Ketoacidosis
FTT	Failure to Thrive
HDN	Haemolytic Disease of the Newborn
HSP	Henoch Schlonein Purpura
IBS	Inflammatory Bowel Disease
MMR	Measles Mumps Rubella (vaccine)
PEFR	Peak Expiratory Flow Rate

PSYCHIATRY

GENERAL PSYCHIATRY HISTORY

History

NOTEPAD

Nature
Onset
Timing
Exacerbating factors (alcohol)
Progression
Associated
Disability

Social

How are things at home? Are there any kids at home?

Extra

Alcohol   Do you drink alcohol?
Drugs   Did you take recreational drugs?
Social   Who's at home with you? Are you supported?

ICE

Ideas   What made you feel this way? Have you had any recent stress?
Concerns   Is there anything you are worried about?
Expectations What do you hope we can do for you today / is there anything
in particular for us to do for you today?

Investigation

Collateral History + MSE
Physical Examination
Rating Scale
Risk Assessment – short, medium and long term & deliberate/non-deliberate
risk

Management

Reassurance and support
Principles of management include a bio-psycho-social approach in the context of
an MDT
Safeguard vulnerable minors
Offer support groups

ADHD

DSM-5: Needs to have happened in 2 settings, for 6 months before age 7: Inattention, Hyperactivity and Impulsiveness

History

Inattention
Easily distracted
Forgetful
Loses things

Hyperactivity
Fidgety
Restless

Impulsiveness
Interrupts others
Can't wait in turn
Blurts out answers

2 settings
Does this happen in school?
Does this happen at home?

Investigation

Same as depression
Rating Scale – **Conner's Questionnaire** & **Strengths and Difficulties Questionnaire**

Management

Specialist referral and assessment

Mild	Parent training and education programmes - watchful waiting for 10 weeks then refer to **CAMHS** or child psychiatrist or paediatrician and medicate – involve MDT
Moderate	CBT + Medical treatment:

Moderate
1st   Methylphenidate (Ritalin) - Monitor growth every 6 months, BP and pulse for pysch disorders
2nd   Atamoxetine
3rd   Dexamphetamine (only if resistant to both 1st & 2nd line)

Severe   Tertiary service and use further combination treatments
Support group - **UK ADHD Partnership (UKAP)**

ALCOHOL

ICD 10: *Drinking Not Problematic Without Three Criteria (need 3/6):*

<u>D</u>esire   <u>W</u>ithdrawal
<u>N</u>eglect   <u>T</u>olerance
<u>P</u>ervasive   <u>C</u>ontrol Lost

History

CAGE – 2/4 then you go into Dependence questions

Do you feel the need to **cut** down?
Do you get **annoyed** when people tell you to drink too much?
Do you feel **guilty** about your drinking?
Is having a drink an **eye-opener** in the morning?

Dependence Questions

Desire (Compulsion)   Do you ever really crave a drink?
Neglect   Anything you miss out on without alcohol?
Pervasive use despite harm   Has alcohol caused you any problems or
                                         difficulties?
Withdrawal   What happens when you don't drink alcohol?
Tolerance   Do you drink more than you used to, to get the
                                         same effect?
Control Lost   Do you feel you've lost control of your
drinking?

Risk Factors

Have you tried to kill yourself before?
Have you been to a psychiatrist before?
Do you have anyone you can talk to?

TRAP Q's
Type
Route
Amount
Pattern (frequency)

Investigation

Blood – FBC (MCV) LFT, B12, folate, U&E, clotting screen (PT, albumin), glucose (hypo)
Blood Alcohol Level
UDS
Rating Scale – **FAST** and **AUDIT** (follows on from CAGE), Severity of Alcohol Dependence Questionnaire (**SADQ**)

Management

Reassurance and support groups – **Alcoholics Anonymous**
Goal: abstinence

Acute Detox   Admit if risk of DT or seizures – involve MDT
Descending regime of Chlordiazepoxide + Pabrinex (thiamine
B1)

Consider **Motivational Interviewing** – if they think they don't
have problems

Long Term   Self-help groups - Alcoholics Anonymous (12 step programme)
Psychological therapies – CBT
Medication – Disulfiram (prevents relapse), Acamprosate (stops
craving)

AUTISM

*ICD10: occurs before age of 3. Impaired **social** interactions, impaired **communication**, and restricted/**repetitive** pattern of behaviour/interests. 1 in 100 – 4 times more boys.*

History

Social Interactions
How is his interaction with other children?
Does he play on his own?
Does he have problems making eye contact?
What do the teachers say about him?

Language
Do you have any concerns about hearing or language?
Does he take words or phrases literally?

Restricted/Repeated
Is there a particular toy or toys he likes playing with?
Does he like a certain routine?
Does he have unusual interests?
How does he react to change?

Asperger's
Does he like memorising timetables or long lists?

Development

Gross	Sits unsupported (**9 months**) walk (**18 months**)
Vision and Fine Motor	Pincer grip (**12 months**), transfer objects between his hands (**9months**)
Hearing and Speech	Three or four words (**12 months**), any concerns about his hearing?
Social and Behaviour	Smile (**10 weeks**) spoon (**18 months**)

Investigation

Hearing test, speech and language assessment, neuropsychological testing (IQ)
Rating Scale – Childhood Autism Rating Scale (**CARS**)

Management

Support and advice from family – **National Autistic Society** and **PORTAGE**

Specialist referral and assessment

Behavioural	Parent training and education programmes.
	Educational approaches - TEACCH
Moderate	CBT + Medical treatment:

	1st	Risperidone (aggression, tantrums and self-injury)
	2nd	Methylphenidate (attention difficulties and hyperactivity)
	3rd	Melatonin (sleep problems)

Severe   Tertiary service and use further combination treatments

EATING DISORDERS

ICD10: more common in females. Poor prognosis. High suicide rates.

Anorexia Nervosa
BMI <17.5 or 15% less than expected
Morbid dread of fatness
Weight losing behaviours
Endocrine

Bulimia Nervosa
BMI>17.5
Morbid dread of fatness
Binging
Purging

History

SCOFF → if 2 or more = eating disorder
Do you make yourself **sick** because you feel uncomfortably full?
Do you worry you've lost **control** over how much you eat
Have you lost more than **one stone** in the last 3 months?
Do you believe you're too **fat** when others say you're too thin?
Does **food** dominate your life?

Eating
How much weight have you lost? Over what period of time?
Do you happen to know your weight and height?
What is your target weight?
Do you avoid certain foods?
Have you ever made yourself throw up?

Physical
Do you exercise?
Do you take substances to make you lose weight?
Do you get periods?

> **Admit if:**
> - BMI <13.5
> - Significant suicide risk
> - Severe sequelae of starvation and purging

Mood
How do you feel about the way you look?
Do you have a fear of gaining wait?
Depression Screen - Do you ever feel low or losing energy?

Risk
Do you think you've lost a significant amount of weight?
Do you feel you need help?

Investigation

Physical exam – including weight and height, lanugo hair, BP, squat test
Bloods and UDS –   **LOW**: ESR, Hb, Plt, WCC, Na, K, Ph, T4   **HIGH**: Glucose, GH, Cortisol, Cholesterol, LFT
ECG – bradycardia, arrhythmia and prolonged QT
DEXA – osteoporosis (if more than 2 year history)
Rating Scale – **Eating Attitudes Test**

Management

Specialist referral and assessment.
Support group - **Beat Eating Disorders (BEAT)**

Psychiatric	Advice on balanced diet, laxatives and diuretics. Negotiate target weight. Refer to dietician and OT.
Anorexia	Self-help and family therapy, MDT
Bulimia	CBT, family therapy, interpersonal therapy and SSRI (Fluoxetine)

BIPOLAR/MANIA

ICD 10: *1 week. Around 1% of population.*

History
Core + Biological **(ASS)** + Cognitive **(MSC)**

Appetite
Sleep
Sex   Are you more active than usual? Are you practicing safe sex?
Memory   Are you more productive than you've ever been?
Spending   Are you spending more money than usual?
Concentration

Depression   Have you been feeling low? You're feeling quite high right now, have you ever felt really low?

Psychotic
Delusions   Do you have any special powers or abilities that others don't have (paranoid/grandiose)?
Hallucinations Has someone famous spoken to you recently?

Risk
Harm   Any thoughts harming yourself? Have you been in trouble recently? What happens when people irritate you?
Suicide   Any thoughts of ending your life?

Extra
Alcohol   Do you drink alcohol?
Drugs   Did you take recreational drugs?
Social   Who's at home with you? Are you supported?

Investigation

1. Collateral History
2. Physical Examination
3. Blood – FBC, TSH (thyroid), LFT (for starting treatment), ECG (lithium)
4. Urine – UDS (drugs)
5. Rating Scale – **Young Mania Rating Scale**
6. Risk assessment

Management

Safeguard vulnerable minors

1st	Admit and record suicidal ideation
2nd	Stop antidepressant
3rd	Consider atypical antipsychotic (olanzapine), if not sleeping BDZ (Lorazepam)
4th	If resistant then give Lithium → monitor LFT and Renal Function
If serious acute	Lorazepam, Haloperidol, Olanzapine

Also consider CBT, MDT and psychoeducation

Support groups - **MIND** and **Bipolar UK**

DELIRIUM

ICD 10: <6 months. 15-20% of all admissions
1. *Impaired consciousness and attention*
2. *Perceptual or cognitive disturbance*
3. *Sudden onset and fluctuates*
4. *Underlying physical cause*

Causes – (DIMTOP)
Drugs (steroids, alcohol)
Infection (UTI)
Metabolic (thyroid, adrenal)
Trauma
Oxygen
Poisoning

History

NOTEPAD

Nature	Tell me what happened (Read entry and the notes)?
	Consciousness & attention?
Onset	When did this first start? Sudden?
Timing	Does you fluctuate? Worse at night (sundowning)?
Exacerbations	Alcohol, drugs, infection (DIMTOP)
Progression	Fluctuates consciousness
Associated	**Perceptions** - Hallucinations, illusions and macropsia/micropsia?
	Thought – delusions
Disability	**Sleep** – do you have difficulty sleeping?

Social

Alcohol	Do you drink alcohol?
Drugs	Did you take recreational drugs?
Social	Who's at home with you? Are you supported?

Investigation

Collateral history + MSE + MMSE
Physical examination – neuro and infection, trauma
Blood - FBC (anemia) white cells, neutrophils, CRP, ESR (infection) U&E (dehydration) blood glucose (DM) TSH (thyroid) LFT (uremia) Ca (Hypercalcemia), Folate and B12, VDRL (syphilis)
Urine Dip + MSU
If indicated - CXR

Management

Preventative
1. Maximise orientation – sensory impairments, clear signage, clocks, calendar and clear lighting, and staff explaining who they are

2. Prevention – decrease polypharmacy, decrease constipation and dehydration, avoid catheters, assess O2 sats and hypoxia
3. Promotion of wellbeing – encourage mobilisation, good pain control, sleep hygiene, healthy diet, social interaction

Treatment

Treat underlying cause

Step up approach:

1. Talk them down
2. Isolate, treat them in a side room
3. Treat with medications (Oral then IM) –
   a. If distressed – ST BDZ (Lorazepam) **or** ST Antipsychotics (Haloperidol, Risperidone) - ECG monitoring → long QT Haloperidol
   b. If alcohol – LT BDZ (Chlordiazepoxide or diazepam)

DEMENTIA

ICD 10: *Acquired, progressive, irreversible global impairment >6 months.*
2.5% of over 70, 20% of over 85 year old

1. *Multiple cognitive defects (memory, language, attentions and cognition)*
2. *Impaired ADL (washing, dressing, handling money)*
3. *Clear consciousness*

History

MMSE	
Mild	25-20
Moderate	20 – 10
Severe	<10

NOTEPAD

Nature	-
Onset	Progressive, >6 months, >60
Timing	Does not fluctuate, day night reversal
Exacerbating Factors	-
Progression	Continuous, irreversible, stepwise (VD)
Associated	Anxiety, depression
Disability	ADL, sleep disturbance

Alzheimer's Disease – (MOLD PPR)

Memory	How is your memory? (AD)
Orientation	Do you ever get lost or wander off? (AD)
Language	Do you have difficulty talking or understanding?
Depression	How is you mood? How is your energy?
Praxis	Do you have difficulty dressing/cooking?
Personality	Has anyone said your personality has changed?
Recognise	Do you have difficulty recognising people or things?

Parkinson's Disease Dementia/Lewy Body Dementia– (BRT)

Bradykinesia
Rigidity
Tremor

Psychotic

Delusions	Have you had any troubling thoughts?
Hallucinations	Have you seen/heard anything others can't hear/see? (LBD)

Risk

Harm	Are you worried about accidentally hurting yourself?

Extra

PMH	DM, stroke, hypertension
Alcohol	Do you drink alcohol?
Social	Who's at home with you? Are you supported?

Investigation

Assessing cognition AMTS, then MMSE, then Addenbrooke's Cognitive Examination (**ACE-R**)

Delirium screen

Neuroimaging – **CT/MRI** (not MRI if pacemaker), **SPECT** (shows how your organs works - LBD 100% specific)

Management- *I assessed all global domains and found... (Exclude other pathologies)*

Reassurance & Support – **Age UK, Old Age Psychiatry Community Team**
Community team and MDT
Refer to memory service
Follow up

Alzheimer's Disease

Home care, day centre, intermittent respite organised by social services, group activities, adaptations at home

Mild – Moderate	AChE inhibitor (Donezepil, Galantamine, Rivastigmine)
Moderate - Severe	NMDA Antagonist (Memantine)
	Severe may require nursing home facilities or carer

Parkinson's Disease Dementia

Symptomatic treatment – no antipsychotics with Parkinsonism

| **1st** | Levodopa (Carbidopa), Dopamine agonist L DOPA), MAOI (Phenelzine) |
| **2nd** | AChE Inhibitors (Donezepil, Galantamine, Rivastigmine), Glutamate agonist (Amantadine) |

Lewy Body Dementia

Symptomatic treatment – no antipsychotics with Parkinsonism

Hallucinations/confusion	AChE inhibitor
Movement	Levodopa (worsens hallucinations – monitor)
Depression	Antidepressants
Sleep disturbance	Clonazepam

DEPRESSION

ICD 10: *2 weeks*

Mild (2 core, 2 other)
Moderate (2 core, 5-6 total)
Severe (3 core, 7 total OR psych OR suicide)

History

Core + Biological **(ASS)** + Cognitive **(GMC)**
Appetite
Sleep
Sex
Guilt
Memory
Concentration

Psychotic

Delusions	Have you had any troubling thoughts (paranoid/nihilistic)?
Hallucinations	Have you seen or heard anything which others can't hear/see?

Risk

Harm	Any thoughts harming yourself?
Suicide	Any thoughts of ending your life?

Extra

PMHx	You're feeling quite low right now, do you ever feel overly high or energetic?
Alcohol	Do you drink alcohol?
Drugs	Did you take recreational drugs?
Social	Who's at home with you? Are you supported?

Investigation

1. Collateral History
2. Physical Examination
3. Blood – FBC (Anaemia), TSH (thyroid), U&E (dehydrated)
4. Urine – Urine dip (DM), UDS (drugs)
5. Rating Scale – **PHQ** (GP) **HADS** (hospital) **CDI** (child)
6. Risk Assessment

Management

Safeguard vulnerable minors
Reassure (25% of population)

Mild   Watchful waiting 2 weeks + monitor patient + give NICE 2010
       Stepped Care Model (home-CBT management therapy)

Moderate   CBT or Citalopram (SSRI) – under 30 follow up in 1 week,
       otherwise 2 weeks (in 8 weeks no response, increase dose)

Severe Augment with Lithium (treatment resistant), ECT

Psychotic   Atypical antipsychotic

Support groups - **MIND** and **Depression Alliance**

GENERALISED ANXIETY DISORDER

ICD 10/DSM5:   *Excessive anxiety or worry occurring most days 6 months, 3-5% prevalence*

4 symptoms: *Autonomic (Palpitations, sweating, trembling, shaking)*
Chest or Abdominal (SOB, pain)
Mental health (psych)
General (flushes, tension)

Management

Rating Scale – **GAD2 Screening Tool**

Reassurance and support – **Anxiety UK**
Safeguard vulnerable minors
Empowerment, communication and wider support

NICE Stepwise Approach in Bio-Psycho-Social:

Step 1   Education and active monitoring
Step 2   Low intensity psychiatric interventions (self-help/psycho-educational groups)
Step 3   High intensity psychiatric interventions (CBT/ applied relaxation), OR
SSRI (Sertraline)/SNRI (Venaflaxine)
Step 4   Highly stepped input – Combination Therapy in Multiagency Team

EXAM POINTS
• Consider organic differentials
• Rule out depression, OCD and psychosis
• Make diagnosis of anxiety disorder
• Discuss psych and pharm therapies
• Know side effects of SSRIs
• Discuss support as carer, self-help groups and charities

MENTAL STATE EXAMINATION

- Appearance and behaviour
  - o Dress
  - o Build
  - o Eye contact and paralanguage
  - o Kempt
- Speech
  - o Rate
  - o Tone
  - o Volume
- Emotion (affect and mood)
  - o Subjective
  - o Objective
- Thought
  - o Delusions
    - ▪ Persecutory
    - ▪ Grandiose
    - ▪ Reference
  - o Thought
    - ▪ Thought insertion, withdrawal and broadcast
  - o Passivity
- Perception
  - o Illusion
  - o Hallucinations
- Cognition
  - o Orientated to time place and person
- Insight
  - o Do they know they are not well?
- Risk Assessment
  - o Harm to self
  - o Harm to others
  - o Harm from others

OBSESSIVE COMPULSIVE DISORDER

ICD 10: *2 weeks. 1% of population*

1. *Acknowledge patient in own mind*
2. *Repetitive and unpleasant (must not be pleasurable) – excessive and unreasonable*
3. *Unable to resist*

History

SEDATED

Symptoms of anxiety	**Physical** - SOB? Palpitations? Nervous?
	Psychological – can you relax and switch off?
Episodic or continuous	Do you always feel like this or some of the time?
	Anankastic - Set order, Meticulous, Perfectionist?
Drink and drugs	Sometimes when people feel stressed they use alcohol or drugs to relieve yourself?
Avoidance and escape	Are there things you avoid because they make you too anxious (work/relationships)?
Timing and triggers	When did these problems start? What made you decide to talk about this today?
Effect on life	How does it affect you (work/relationships)?
Depression	How has your mood been? How is your energy?

OCD Specific

Obsession	Are your thoughts your own thoughts? Do you have any recurrent or intrusive thoughts?
Compulsion	How do you make them go away (make them give examples)? Does it make you feel calmer? Do you feel like you can resist these actions?
Perception	Do you hear or see anything which other people can't see or hear?
Insight	Do you think this is unreasonable or excessive or do you think this is normal?

ICE

Ideas	What made you feel this way? Have you had any recent stress?
Concerns	Is there anything you are worried about?

Expectations   What do you hope we can do for you today / is there anything in particular for us to do for you today?

Investigation

Blood – organise causes - FBC, TSH,
Rating Scale – **Yale Brown OCD**

Management

Reassurance and support – **OCD UK**
Safeguard vulnerable minors
Empowerment, communication and wider support

Mild	CBT (Brief Individual or Group)
Moderate	CBT or SSRI (Citalopram/Fluoxetine)
Severe	CBT and SSRI → give TCA is resistant (Clomipramine)

OVERDOSE

History

Story

Act	Tell me what happened? How long ago was it?
Trigger	Was there anything that triggered this?
Degree of Planning	How long were you planning this? Did you put your affairs in order before hand?
Precautions	did you do anything to prevent people interrupting you
Method	How many tablets did you take? Did you take any alcohol or anything with it?
Purpose	did you hope this will kill you
Discovery	Were you found or did you get help? How do you feel about that?

Now

Regret	Do you regret trying to kill yourself?
Wishes	Do you still wish you were dead?
Symptoms	Abdo pain, vomiting

Future

Future	How do you see the future?
Help seeking	Would you like help with the stress you're experiencing?

Risk Factors

Have you tried to kill yourself before?
Have you been to a psychiatrist before?
Do you have anyone you can talk to?

Psychotic

Delusions	Have you had any troubling thoughts?
Hallucinations	Have you seen or heard anything which others can't hear/see?

Extra

Depression screen   How has your mood been? How is your energy?
Current drugs/ alcohol
Relationship problems

Investigation

Rating Scale – **Columbia Suicide Severity Rating Scale**

Physical examination – pupils, resp, abdo, neuro, cardio

IV access – bloods paracatamol levels (4 hrs post), LFT, INR, FBC, glucose, ABG, ECG (potentially), CT (neuro signs)

Normogram – graph for plotting paracetamol levels and see the need to treat under the line → >12g could be fatal

TOXBASE – look up antidotes. For more help contact **UK National Poisons Information Centre**

Management

Physical treatment

ABCDE + IV Access + glucose + NAC infusion (paracetamol)

Involve specialist in psych assessment

Immediate Interventions

Mild/ Medium Risk	Try home management, take problem solving approach, make a plan to deal with future suicidal ideation and thoughts of self-harm – including how they get hold of drugs
High Risk	Admit into psychiatric
LFT	Show acute fulminant liver failure – go to ICU
Acidotic	Consider dialysis

Treat underlying psychiatric condition (consider low toxicity antidepressant – SSRI)

Long Term Inteventions

Follow up within a week – via community mental health team (outpatients) OR GP + CBT

Crisis resolution team - support at home, operate 24hrs and see people 2 times daily

Assertive outreach Team (OAT) – intensive treatment and support in the community → to assure treatment

Support group – **Samaritans** and **PAPYRUS** (children and adolescent)

POSTNATAL DEPRESSION

ICD 10: 1st month, peaks 3rd month. Baby blues (70-80%), depression (10%) →
most resolve in 6 months.

History

Core + Biological (ASS) + Cognitive (GMC)

Appetite
Sleep
Sex
Guilt
Memory
Concentration

Baby (TBH PC)

Thoughts	How do you feel towards the baby? Is there anything particularly frightening you?
Bonding	Are you bonding? Are you breastfeeding?
Hurt	Have you had any thoughts of harming your baby?
Planned	Was the baby planned?
Children	Are there any other children at home?

Psychotic

Delusions	Have you had any troubling thoughts?
Hallucinations	Have you seen or heard anything which others can't hear/see?

Risk

Harm	Any thoughts harming yourself?
Suicide	Any thoughts of ending your life?

Social

Alcohol	Do you drink alcohol? Did you drink during your pregnancy?
Drugs	Did you take recreational drugs in pregnancy?
Social	Who's at home with you? Are you supported? How do your friends describe you (Premorbidity)?

ICE

Ideas	What made you feel this way? Have you had any recent stress?
Concerns	Is there anything you are worried about?

Expectations   What do you hope we can do for you today / is there anything in particular for us to do for you today?

Investigation

Same as depression
Rating Scale – Edinburgh Postnatal Depression Scale (**EDPS**)

Management

Reassurance & Support – **Pre And Post Natal Depression Advice & Support**
                                        (**PANDAS**)
Empowerment, communication and wider support
Safeguard vulnerable minors

Mild – Moderate	Facilitated Self-help Strategies, with support practitioner (Home CBT)
Moderate – Severe	CBT (all)
	SSRI - Paroxetine (if declined psych therapy/failure)
	Mother Baby Unit (if severe or children are at home – ensuring safe environment)
	ECT (if very severe)

POST-TRAUMATIC STRESS DISORDER

ICD 10: *Within 6 months, diagnosis is at 1 month. Experiencing 4 months.*

History

PTSD Specific – (**HATER**)

Hyperarousal	Do you feel on edge or jumpy?
Avoidance	Are there certain things/situations you can't face since this has happened?
Trauma	When did it start? I know it's difficult for you to talk about, but could you tell me what happened please? Were you badly hurt? Did you see someone else got hurt?
Emotional Numbing	Do you feel numb?
Re-experiencing	Have you had any flashbacks? Or bad dreams/nightmares?

SEDATED

Symptoms of anxiety	**Physical** - SOB? Palpitations? Nervous? **Psychological** – can you relax and switch off?
Episodic or continuous	Do you always feel like this or some of the time?
Drink and drugs	Sometimes when people feel stressed they use alcohol or drugs to relieve yourself?
Avoidance and escape	Are there things you avoid because they make you too anxious (work/relationships)?
Timing and triggers	
Effect on life	How does it affect you (work/relationships)?
Depression	How has your mood been? How is your energy?

Investigation

Rating Scale – **HADS** & clinician administered PTSD Scale for DSM5 (**CAPS 5**)

Management

Reassurance and support – **MIND**
Safeguard vulnerable minors
Empowerment, communication and wider support

Treatment:

< 4 weeks	Watchful waiting
> 4 weeks	1st - trauma focused CBT or Eye Movement Desensitisation and Reprocessing (EMDR)
	2nd - SSRI (Paroxetine)/ NASSA (Mirtazapine)
>12 weeks	TCA (Imipramine/Amytriptalline)

If can't sleep – consider Lorazepam

PSYCHOSIS

ICD 10: 1 month. Losing touch with reality, experience hallucinations and delusions. 1 symptom of First Rank (Panic At the Disco) OR 2 of Second Rank

History

Panic At The Disco

Passivity — Do you have full control of everything you do and feel?

Auditory Hallucinations — Do you ever hear anything that other people can't?

Thought Interference — Do you feel you're in control of your thoughts?
Do you ever feel other people know what you're thinking?

Delusions of Perception — Have you ever received a sign which has meant something to you?

Negative symptoms

Depression — 3 core

Social Withdrawal — Do you find you're spending more time by yourself and less time with others?

Delusions — Do you think anyone is out there to harm you in anyway (paranoid)?

Conviction — Sometimes people's minds play tricks on them when they're stress – do you think this is the case?

Risk

Harm — Did the thoughts or voices ever tell you to harm yourself or others around you?

Suicide — Do you have any thoughts of ending your life?

Extra

Alcohol — Do you drink alcohol?

Drugs — Did you take recreational drugs?

Social — Who's at home with you? Are you supported?

Investigation

Collateral History

Physical Examination
Blood – FBC (clozapine weekly), U&E, lipids and LFT (before antipsych), VDRL (syphilis), CT (if organic suspected)
Urine – UDS (drugs)
Rating Scale – **Brief Psychiatric Rating Scale**
Assess status – ADL assessment and housing and financy

Management

Safeguard vulnerable minors

Acute

Early Intervention Service (EIS) – to minimise the duration of untreated psychosis to 3 months (provide psychoeducation and reduce relapse)
Antipsychotics (olanzapine) - use Depot (Risperidone/ Flupentixol) if compliance issues

Reduce Relapse + LT

Family therapy (decrease expressed emotion), concordance therapy, art therapy
Psychological CBT (gain insight)

Support Help employment, study, benefits and groups: **SANE** and **MIND**

AMTS QUESTIONNAIRE

AMTS screening tool (MY ARAB WELT)

<u>M</u>onarch
<u>Y</u>ear

<u>A</u>ddress (ask patient to memorise an address e.g. 42 West Street)
<u>R</u>ecognise person
<u>A</u>ge
<u>B</u>irthday

<u>W</u>W1 date
<u>E</u>numeration
<u>L</u>ocation
<u>T</u>ime

Do you remember the **address** I gave you?

Hodgkinson AMTS Scoring:

Mild	<7
Moderate	4-6
Severe	0-3

GENERAL GYNAECOLOGY HISTORY

History

Symptoms – 4 P's

Pain	Shoulder tip pain (ectopic)? Cyclical? During sex?
PV bleed	When? After sex?
PV discharge	Amount? Colour? Smell? Blood?
Pregnant	Have you ever been pregnant? How many children? Delivery? Complications? Birth weight?

Menstruation

LMP?
Regularity?
Heaviness?
How many pads?
Flooding – night? Clots? Tampon + pad?

Red flags   PCB, PMB. IMB

> **If fertility problems:**
> - How often having sex?
> - Either partner w/previous child?
> - Any mumps history?
> - Any PID/STI history?
> - Does partner work abroad?

Other – (SSC)

Smears	When did you get it done? Was it normal?
Sex	Are you currently sexually active? Have you had any STI's? Dyspareunia?
Contraception	Are you currently on any contraception? What contraception have you used in the past?

Systems – Urine + FLAWS

Urine	Any problems passing urine? (Fibroids/UTI)
FLAWS	
Overall	Check patient's mood and mental health

Investigation

1. Physical Examination   General + abdo exam (tenderness)
   Signs of anaemia (blood loss)
2. Speculum + smear (high vaginal or endocervical) + pH (BV/trichomoniasis)
3. PV exam (position of cervix + dilation)
4. Urine and blood BHCG
5. Bloods – anemia, TSH (thyroid), hormones

AMENNORRHEA

History

Frequency + Duration

Pregnancy

- Sexually active?
- Pregnancy test?
- **Pregnancy symptoms**   morning N+V, breast tender, urinary freq

Hypothalamic Hypogonadism

- Exercise
- Diet (weight loss)
- Stress

Prolactinoma

- Headache
- Visual disturbance (Bitemporal hemianopia)
- Nipple discharge (Galactorrhea)

Thyroid

- Change in bowel habit
- Palpitation
- Tremor

PCOS

- Acne
- Hirsutism
- Weight gain

Premature Ovarian Failure

- Flushes
- Dryness (loss of libido)
- Night sweats

DIFFERENTIALS
• Pregnancy
• Hypothalamic hypogonadism
• Prolactinokma
• Thyroid
• PCOS
• Ovarian failure/ menopause

PCOS
LT implications
Management of anovulation
Bio-psycho-social of Dx
Health promotion and healthy dieting

Investigation

Urinary or serum bHCG

Blood – TFT, prolactin, androgens, oestradiol, gonadotrophins:

Low = hypothalamic   **Raised** = ovarian problem (e.g. Premature ovarian failure)

CONTRACEPTION

History

Patient

Sexual intercourse   When was last sexual intercourse? Condoms?
STD   Ever been to STD clinic or had STD? Did you receive and complete treatment?
Partner   Do you have a regular partner? Have you slept with anyone else in the past three months?
Partner demographic   Gender, age, occupation, how did you meet met?
Gynae history   LMP? Regular? Heavy?

Counselling

Key points:
1. All the contraceptive methods, apart from condoms, do not protect again STI
2. Whenever you have a new sexual partner to have a STI screen 3 weeks and 3 months after unprotected sex
3. Always remember emergency contraception is available from A&E or GP or pharmacy

Gillick Competence:
1. Understand doctor's advice
2. Can't be persuaded to inform their parents
3. Likely to begin intercourse with or without contraception
4. Unless they receive contraception their mental or physical health is likely to suffer
5. It's in their best interest

Investigations

Examination   BMI & BP
Screen   STI screen, refer to GUM clinic

Provide leaflets to patient

Contraception Available:

Type	Pill Name	PI	Advantages	Disadvantages
Pills	OCP	0.2%	Effective S/E uncommon Ease painful and heavy periods	Very small risk of clots Nausea, headache Must remember to take it
	POP	1%	Less chance of serious	Must take it same time daily Irregular periods
Implants	Nexplanon	<1%	Very effective	Periods become irregular S/E – weight gain and spots
Injection	Depo-Provera/ Noristerat	<1%	Very effective Don't need to remember to take	24 months return fertility Osteoporosis
Coils	IUD	<0.5%	Very effective Don't need to remember to take	Periods heavier or painful
	IUS	<0.2%	Very effective Don't need to remember to take Reduces bleeding	Unpredictable bleeding S/E – weight gain and spots
Barrier	Condoms	2-15%	Protects against STI	Have to remember to wear

ECTOPIC PREGNANCY

1% of all pregnancies. 95% in fallopian tube.

History

Symptoms – 4 P's

Pain	Cyclical? Colicky (ectopic), shoulder tip pain (ectopic), diarrhoea
PV bleed	When? Prune red colour, clotting, and amount?
PV discharge	Amount? Colour? Smell? Blood?
Pregnant	Have you ever been pregnant? How many children?

Delivery? Complications? Birth weight?

Menstruation

LMP?

Regularity?

Heaviness? How many pads? Flooding – especially at night? Clots? Tampon + pad?

Other – (SSC)

Smears	When did you get it done? Was it normal?
Sex	Are you currently sexually active? Have you had any STI's? Dyspareunia?
Contraception	Are you currently on any contraception? What contraception have you used in the past?
Risk factors	Infections, trauma, age, alcohol, smoking, drugs
PMH	DM, connective tissue disease, uterine abnormalities

Patient care – WHO's

Who's at home with you? Any other support? How is everything at home? Who is in charge of your care? (Midwife/consultant)

Overall – check patient's mood and mental health

Investigation

ABC assess if haemodynamically stable

Examination	Tachycardia, abdo pain + rebound cervical excitation, OS closed, uterus smaller than dates
Investigations	Serum & urine, USS, FBC, Rh, cross match

Management

Acute	Haemo unstable - low BP, high HR, live bleeding ectopic):
	2 large bore (grey) cannulae + Nil by mouth
	Bloods taken. Group & save. IV fluids
	Give Anti D
	Salpingectomy on laparotomy → 15% HCG drop in 4 days
	otherwise methotrexate
Subacute	Haemo stable
Conservative	HCG<1000 - repeat HCG 48hrs
Medical	HCG<3000 & no cardiac activity 4-5wks
	Methotrexate → If no 15% drop in 4 days then 2nd dose.
Surgical	HCG>3000
	Laparascopic salpingostomy (preserves fertility better) or
	salpingectomy

All serial HCG until <20

GENERAL SEXUAL HISTORY

History

Patient – 4 Q's
When was last sexual intercourse? Condoms?
Ever been to STD clinic or had STD? Did you receive and complete treatment?
Do you have a regular partner? Have you slept with anyone else in the past
three months?
Any recent travel?

Partner – 6 Q's
Nationality
Male or female
Concerns about his/her sexual health
Type of intercourse – vaginal, anal, oral? Give or receive?
HIV status?
Does he have symptoms?

PMH
Diabetes mellitus (candida)

DH
OCP (discharge)
Antibiotic use
Blood transfusion
Illicit drugs – IV drugs? Sharing needles?

Investigation

Examination	Tenderness, cervical excitation (PID)
Swab	**High Vaginal** – BV, candida, trochomonas
	Endocervical – chlamydia, gonorrhoea
Urinary	BHCG, urine dip (leukocyte and coliform – UTI), urinary PCR (chlamidya)
Blood	Syphilis, gonorrhoea, HIV

SMEAR

History

SSC

Smears	When did you get it done? Was it normal?
Sex	Are you currently sexually active? Have you had any STI's? Dyspareunia?
Contraception	Are you currently on any contraception? What contraception have you used in the past?

Counselling

Smear	Introduce, check patient details. Offer chaperone and wash hands and wear gloves. I'd like to perform a speculum examination today. Have you had one before? It will involve me inserting an instrument called a speculum (show to patient) in your vagina and taking some samples around the neck of your womb. Would that be alright? I'll need you to undress yourself from the waist downwards and lay on the couch (flattened). Can you now bring your heels towards your bottom and let your knees fall apart. You can cover yourself with this blanket.
Prepare	Smear sample pot: unscrew lid and label with pt name, date of birth, NHS no. and today's date. On form record LMP (smear best done mid cycle) and whether on OCP. Prepare light source for visualisation of cervix. Apply KY lubricating jelly to the side of Cusco speculum. Are you experiencing any pain?
Inspect	Outer vagina: skin changes, lesions, redness, swelling. Use your left hand to part the labia and tell the patient 'I'm now going to insert the speculum.' Insert speculum with screw facing sideways, rotating it upwards as you advance it. Fix the screw to secure the speculum. Use cytobrush and rotate clockwise 5 times inside the cervix. Tap inside the smear pot 10 times and then dispose cytobrush. Re-screw the smear pot lid. Unscrew speculum

and remove speculum gently, ensuring you do not catch the cervix as you withdraw it.

'Thank you, you can now get dressed again.'

Smear Examination

Examination	Introduce, check pt details, wash hands, offer chaperone. Ask if any pain and offer to explain procedure: I'd like to examine your tummy and check how baby is doing today. Would that be alright? I'll need you to lay on your back on the couch (45 degrees) and lift your top up for me please.
Inspection	Linea nigra Scars Fetal movements Striae gravidarum Bruising (self-administered LMWH) Distension (consistent with pregnancy)
Palpation	SFH – do three times (take average, remove outlier) blinded and from pubis symphysis to fundus (feel with ulnar edge of hand) **Model is always 34cm SFH – Note the gestation on candidate brief, and consider whether LGA SGA**
Palpate Fetus	*Tip: Fetal head feels a lot harder than bottom. Keep one hand stationary, and feel with the other and vice versa* Lie: Longitudinal/Transverse/Oblique (fetal spine on maternal left/right). Presentation: Cephalic/Breech. **Models are usually not engaged** (minimum 3/5ths palpable). Use Pawlik's grip if needed, otherwise use flats of fingers from both hands.
Auscultate FHR	Using ultrasound transducer (Sonicaid) or Pinard stethoscope over anterior shoulder (between head and umbilicus). If using Pinard, place with hand, and put your ear on the Pinard, with hands behind your back. Present lie, presentation, SFH, engagement and FHR if measured. Present findings as you do the examination.
To complete	Check basic observations (HR/RR/Temp/BP/O2 sat) and urine dipstick (protein/leukocytes/nitrites).

TERMINATION

History (ICE)

Ideas	I can see that this is very difficult for you right now. Have you had any thoughts on whether you'd like to keep this pregnancy? Why do you want the termination? Have you any ideas of keeping the baby?
Concerns	I understand that you are considering an abortion. Do you have any particular worries or concerns about this? Have you given this decision much thought? Do you wish to speak to someone before you make a decision? Who's at home with you? Any other support? How is everything at home?
Expectations	What would you like us to do for your today?

Obstetric History

How many weeks are you so far?

How many pregnancies/children previously?

How was baby conceived? Planned or unplanned pregnancy? How do you feel about that?

Any complications?

Sexual History

Sexual intercourse	When was last sexual intercourse? Condoms?
STD	Ever been to STD clinic or had STD? Did you receive and complete treatment?
Partner	Do you have a regular partner? Have you slept with anyone else in the past three months?
Partner demographic	Gender, age, occupation, how did you meet met?

Gynaecology History

LMP? Regular? Heavy? Length?

Investigation

Examination	Tenderness, cervical excitation (PID)
Swab	**High vag** – BV, candida, trochomonas OR
	Endocervical – chlamidya, gonorrhoea
Urinary	BHCG, urine dip, urinary PCR (chlamidya)
Blood	Syphilis, gonorrhoea, HIV
Examination	Tenderness, cervical excitation (PID)

Counselling

Explaining

Accessibility	State that the service is free under the National Health Service.
Confidentiality	Reassure the patient that the procedure will remain confidential.
Appointments	Explain that she will be given two separate appointments. The fi rst, to assess eligibility and choice of procedure; the second will be the procedure itself. Also mention that the abortion should be completed within 3 weeks of the fi rst contact she has made with the services

Option 1

"I understand that you wish to proceed with the abortion. I would like to explain the different options available. The first option is to abort the pregnancy using tablets. You will be given a tablet called mifepristone which stops the pregnancy hormones from working and makes you have an early miscarriage. A few days after this you will be given another tablet that can be taken by mouth or inserted into the vagina, which will cause the pregnancy to be expelled. This option is 99% successful if used before 8 weeks and must be carried out before the pregnancy has reached 9 weeks."

Option 2

"The second option is a minor surgical procedure which is usually performed before the pregnancy has reached its 12th week. You will not need to be put to sleep since it will be done under local anaesthetic.
A small tube will be passed into the womb and the pregnancy will be removed. This is a fairly quick procedure and should only take 5 minutes."

Option 3

"After 12 weeks of pregnancy, a more extensive surgical procedure is required. This involves putting you to sleep under general anaesthetic and removing the pregnancy through a tube passed into your womb.
You may need to stay overnight in the hospital after the procedure has been carried out."

Potential Complications   There may be complications associated with termination
- Heavy bleeding
- Damage to the cervix or womb
- Minimal chance of affecting fertility
- Failure to terminate the pregnancy, requiring further treatment

Rhesus status   If necessary anti-D injection may need to be administered

STD Screen   Explain to the patient that all women attending for an abortion are screened for chlamydia to reduce the chances of post-operation infection (salpingitis)

Implications   Discuss with the patient possible implications after having the abortion, such as her fertility not being compromised and possible emotional response.

Fertility: 'It is important to appreciate that having a successful abortion will not compromise your future chances of falling pregnant.'

Counsellor: 'After having an abortion, some women experience a number of different emotions. You may feel relieved or sad. All of this is perfectly natural. If you are having problems coping with your emotions, I can put you in touch with a counsellor, if you feel you need to talk to someone.'

Management

Important: No impact on future fertility.

<9 weeks - Medical: Home

Day 1   Mifepristone 200mg PO (anti progesterone)

Day 3   Misoprostol 600mcg PV (progstaglandin)

IF abortion not occured w/in 4hrs → give another 400mcg of Misoprostol
>22 weeks KCL into umblicial vein

>9 weeks - Medical: admit & treat

Surgical > 7 weeks. PV misoprostol given prior to soften cervix

Suction curettage 7- 13 weeks → suction impossible after 13 weeks

-Dilation & evacuation >13weeks
Surgical is with antibiotic cover
Surgical risk: infection, haemorrhage, perforation

Abortion Act 1967:
A. Risk to life of mum
B. Prevent grave permanent injury to physical or mental health of mum
C. Injury to physical or mental health of mum
D. Injury to physical or mental

Minors

In girls aged under 16 years, form HSA1 must be signed by two doctors. GMC guidelines are that girls <16 years may be able to reach an informed decision depending on their capacity to comprehend everything involved in the procedure. However, in those cases where a competent underage girl refuses termination, it may be possible for a parent or guardian to authorise.

URINARY GYNAE

History

Urinary Symptoms – (FUNDISH BBC DD)

Frequency
Urgency
Nocturia
Dysuria
Incontinence
Suprapubic pain
Haematuria

Back/loin pain (pyelonephritis/neurological)
Bowel symptoms (incontinence, constipation)
Chronic cough (smoker/increase abdo pressure)

Dragging sensation/lump (prolapse)
Diet (coffee, alcohol)

Past Obstetric

Parity	How many pregnancies?
Instrumental	Were any instruments used during delivery?
Prolonged	

PMH

Neurological
Abdominal or pelvic surgery

DH

HRT

Investigation

Examination	Tenderness, cervical excitation (PID)
Urinary diary	Consider if urge incontinence
Swab	**High Vaginal** – BV, candida, trichomonas
	Endocervical – chlamydia, gonorrhoea
Urinary	BHCG, urine dip + MSSU + cystoscopy
Consider	USS (urgency is an indication, menopause to see atrophic ovaries, pressure effects of fibroids) + urodynamics

---

DIFFERENTIALS

- Incontinence
  - Stress 50%
  - Urge 35%
  - Mix 10%
  - Overflow 1%
  - Unknown 4%
- UTI
- Bladder pathology
- Pelvic mass (pressure effects)
- Diabetes

GENERAL OBSTETRIC HISTORY

Ask to all general obs presentations

History

Pregnancy – HOW's
How many weeks pregnant are you?
LMP? Are your periods regular?
How many pregnancies/children?
How was baby conceived? Planned pregnancy?

        If **planned** – congratulate mother
        If **unplanned** - how do you feel about it?

How many are you carrying – Is this a single or multiple pregnancy?
How many scans have you had? (Must have had 2 scans - 10 and 20 weeks)

> **DVT History**
>
> *DVTs are the most common obstetric condition!*
>
> Common symptoms:
> Chest pain
> Shortness of breath
> Haemoptysis
> Leg swelling

Complications – WHAT's
What were your booking blood results – BP, diabetes?
What complications: mum – blurred vision, pain, headache, <u>blood loss</u>, broken waters

                baby – feeling movement? Growth?

Patient care – WHO's
Who's at home with you? Any other support? How is everything at home?
Who is in charge of your care? (midwife/consultant led)

Overall – check patient's mood and mental health

Investigation

1. Physical Examination – General examination, abdominal examination (consider neuro – Pre-ecplampsia)
2. Doppler SonicAid OR Pinard stethoscope
3. Measure symphysis-fundal height (SFH), check engagement (only after 36weeks), check blood pressure and urine dip
4. Consider kick chart – record how many times the baby has kicked (if worried about baby not kicking)
5. Consider USS, Amniocentesis, CVS - depends on gestation

BREATHLESSNESS

DIFFERENTIAL
DVT: musculoskeletal, trauma or dermatological.
PE: chest infection, intra-abdominal bleed.

History

Onset	Acute or chronic?
PE	Dyspnoea, pleuritic chest pain, haemoptysis, faintness, collapse
DVT	Leg pain and discomfort (usually on left side), swelling, tenderness, oedema, fever, abdominal pain
Bleeding	Any bleeding anywhere (anaemia)

Rule out asthma (common) and other causes of breathlessness (cardiac, respiratory)

Assess impact of breathlessness (at rest, mild, moderate or strenuous exertion)

POHx: previous instrumental delivery or C/S, pre-eclampsia, prolonged labour, multiparity

Travel history (>4hr travel)

Risk factors for VTE

Factors Specific to Pregnancy	Inherited	Acquired
Venous stasis	Strong family history	Previous thrombotic
Age ≥35 years	Factor V Leiden mutation	event
Multiparity	(most common)	Obesity
Gestation <36 weeks	Prothrombin gene	Long-haul travel
Instrument-assisted	G20210A mutation	Hormonal Tx (OCP, HRT)
or caesarean delivery	Antithrombin III	Immobilisation
Haemorrhage	deficiency	Cancer
Pre-eclampsia	Protein C deficiency	Trauma
Prolonged labour	Protein S deficiency	IBD
	Hyperhomocysteinaemia	Sepsis + UTI
	Dysfibrinogenaemia	Gross varicose veins
	Disorders of plasminogen and plasminogen activation	APLS
		CVA
		Polycythaemia vera
		Sickle cell disease

Examination

Cardio, abdo exam

Check basic observations – fever, tachypnoea, O2 sats, tachycardia, ABG

Blood - FBC (exclude anaemia, raised WCC in DVT), U&E (exclude dehydration before anticoagulation), coagulation screen

PE   Do CXR and compression duplex US

- o   If normal but clinical suspicion remains → repeat V/Q or CTPA scan
- o   if abnormal → CTPA

     Counselling: gain informed consent. V/Q scan childhood cancer risk higher than CTPA, but CTPA has lower maternal breast cancer risk in mother (less than 1/1,000,000)

DVT   Compression duplex US

- o   If –ve and low suspicion → discontinue Tx
- o   If –ve and high suspicion → repeat scan 1wk later whilst keeping patient anticoagulated

In general, if clinical suspicion remains high despite negative investigation results, you should repeat the tests whilst providing anticoagulation.

Prophylactic Management

- TED stockings for women travelling >4hr or hospitalised pt or pt with contraindication to LMWH.
- Titrate LMWH dose to anti-Factor 10a level.

Antenatal

- Encourage hydration and mobilisation.
- Offer pre-pregnancy counselling and a prospective management plan for thromboprophylaxis in pregnancy.
- If recurrent VTE and on warfarin (teratogenic) already → change to LMWH as early as possible (teach pt how to self-inject [may see abdominal bruising O/E]).
- LMWH antenatally and for 6wk postpartum if:
  - o   Original VTE unprovoked/idiopathic/oestrogen-related/other risk factors/+ve FHx of VTE in 1st degree relative/known thrombophilia.

- Asymptomatic inherited/acquired thrombophilia ONLY → close surveillance antenatally and at least 1 week postpartum prophylaxis.

Intrapartum

- Women on LMWH should alert delivery ward staff when contractions begin/if they bleed vaginally and **stop** injections. Hospital assessment and further doses prescribed by medical staff.
- There is a haemorrhage risk and anaesthetic procedures must be delayed by 24hr since last dose.

Postpartum prophylaxis

- Any previous VTE or anyone requiring antenatal prophylactic LMWH → 6wk LMWH postpartum
- Obese (BMI >40) or emergency C/S → 1wk LMWH postpartum
- If elective C/S plus one or more additional risk factors → 1wk LMWH postpartum
- Consider follow-up in joint obstetric-haematology clinic.

Complications

- Thrombophilia and placental vascular complications: fetal loss, IUGR, HELLP syndrome.
- Post-thrombotic syndrome after DVT.
- Prolonged unfractionated heparin use during pregnancy → osteoporosis and fractures.

GESTATIONAL DIABETES MELLITUS

History

Pregnancy – HOW's

How many weeks are you so far? LMP? Was it regular?
How many pregnancies/children?
How was baby conceived? Planned or unplanned pregnancy? How do you feel about that?
How many scans have you had? (Must have had 2 scans - 10 and 20 weeks)
How has the pregnancy been so far? Any complications?

Obstetric History Qs

Symptoms	Polyuria, polydipsia, weight loss, infections - UTI
Previous	DM & GDM – what were your levels? How was it Tx?
Other	Family history DM, alcohol, smoking

> **Risk Factors GDM**
> Previous stillbirth
> Polyhydramnios
> Glycosuria
> Previous fetus >4.5kg
> Positive FHx
> BMI >30
> Race

Counselling

DM is high sugar in blood – common in pregnancy (2-5%)
GDM usually develops in 3rd trimester, usually disappears after birth, more likely to get DM in later life

Explain risk

Mother - increase infections
Baby - high sugar therefore big baby so increased chance C/S
➔   Good BG control decreases risks

> **WHO Diagnostic Criteria**
> FPG > 5.6
> 75g 1hr OGTT > 7.8

Monitoring

Monitor BP, urinalysis, regular serum creatinine and urea, foetal echo + USS growth 4 weekly + 4 chamber heart view USS at 20 weeks. Deliver at 40 weeks. Screening at booking if previous GDM. If normal repeat at 16 and 28 weeks. Screen at 28 weeks if RFs.

Management

Newly diagnosed women should be seen in a joint diabetes and antenatal clinic within a week

Medication   Fasting BG > 7 mmol/l → insulin should be started
Fasting BG < 7 mmol//l → 2 week diet and exercise:
- Self-monitoring of BG w/glucometer
- Diet - Refer ALL to dietician
- Exercise - 30mins walking/day until just breathless
- Target: Fasting BG - 5.3 but >4 to prevent hypoglycaemia
        1hr BG - 7.8 or 2hr BG - 6.4

If 2 weeks glucose target not met → Metformin
If 2 weeks glucose target not met → Insulin
If metformin intolerant or fail to meet target → Glibenclamide

Preventative Measures Folic acid 5mg + Aspirin from 12 weeks (prevent PET)
Management of pre-existing diabetes   Stop oral agents, apart from metformin, and commence insulin
Weight loss for women with BMI of > 27
Folic acid 5 mg/day from pre-conception to 12 weeks gestation
Rx microvascular (retinopathy) and macrovascular

HIV IN PREGNANCY

2.5 women in 1000. Without intervention 15-45% of babies infected. With intervention <1% babies infected.

History

Pregnancy – HOW's

How many weeks are you so far? LMP? Was it regular? How many pregnancies/children?
How was baby conceived? Planned or unplanned pregnancy? How do you feel about that?
How many scans have you had? (Must have had 2 scans - 10 and 20 weeks)

Partner – 3 Q's

Partner   Regular? Only one? Nationality, male or female, their sexual health, HIV status?
Sex   Are you currently sexually active? Have you had any STI's? Dyspareunia?
Contraception   Are you currently on any contraception? What contraception have you used in the past?

Complications – WHAT's

Infections   STD? Other chest/ skin infections? Travel? Blood transfusions/STD? HIV status?
HIV status   Monitoring results? When did you find out? HIV status of existing children and partner?

Patient care – WHO's

Who's at home with you? Any other support? How is everything at home?
Who is in charge of your care? (Midwife/consultant)
Health promotion for her children and husband

Investigation

HIV screening to all pregnant women at booking
Exam   FBC, LFTs, renal function tests
HIV blood results   Plasma viral load, CD4 lymphocyte count, HIV genotype
Other infections   Hep C screen, HSV, VDRL

Management

To reduce vertical transmission   Maternal antiretroviral therapy
Mode of delivery (caesarean section)
Neonatal antiretroviral therapy
Infant feeding (bottle feeding)

ART	All women offered ART regardless of whether they were taking it or not previously. RCOG guideline recommend starting 28-32 weeks and continued intrapartum
Zidovudine Monotherapy	If viral load is <10,000/ml + if willing to deliver by prelabour caesarean section (PLCS); Started <30 weeks
HAART	If viral load >10,000/ml & no maternal indication for HAART, commenced 22-24 weeks. If multidrug resistance detected **N.B.** HAART is assoc. w/ preterm delivery before 34 weeks
Short-Term Antiretroviral (START)	Prevention of MTCT (mother to child transmission) Discontinued after pregnancy when viral load <50/ml

Delivery   If treated w/ HAART VD recommended if viral load <50 copies/ml at 36 weeks; otherwise CS

ZDV should be started 4 hours before CS

Neonatal ART   ZDV is administered PO to neonate if maternal viral load is <50/ml

Triple ART if viral load >50/ml

Therapy continued for 4-6 weeks

Breast feeding   In UK all women should be advised not to breast feed

HYPEREMESIS GRAVIDARUM

History

Pregnancy – HOW's

How many weeks are you so far? LMP? Was it regular?
How many pregnancies/children?
How was baby conceived? Planned or unplanned pregnancy? How do you feel about that?
How many carrying - single or multiple pregnancies?
How many scans have you had? (Must have had 2 scans - 10 and 20 weeks)

Complications

Symptoms	**Vomit**: duration, frequency, amount, colour (bile) – any blood?
	Chest pain? (Mallory Weiss tear)
	Collapse
	Tremor, palpitations (hyperthyroid)
	FLAWS (check for low Na and K)
	Leg pain, chest pain (DVT/PE)
	Personality changes, forgetfulness (Wernicke Korsakoff)
PMH	Hyperthyroidism? Previous pregnancy? Hyperemesis? Twins
FH?	
FH	Anyone else w/similar problem?

Patient care – WHO's

Who's at home with you? Any other support? How is everything at home?
Who is in charge of your care? (midwife/consultant)

Information

What is it	HG is weight loss >5% w/ketosis. 1st trimester. Unlikely after 12wks. Peaks 6-8wks resolves by 16wks in 90% of women
Causes	Multiple pregnancy, molar pregnancy
Prevalence	80% get N&V in pregnancy. <1% get HG

Investigation

General	Signs of dehydration, BP, HR, Temp
Abdo exam	Appendicitis (guarding + tenderness), large for dates (multiple)
Urine	HCG, Urine dip (ketones, specific gravity - dehydration, nitrites leukocytes - UTI)

Blood	**FBC** - high hct, **U&E** - Low Na + K + urea + alkalosis, **LFT** – high, **TFT** (high transient resolves by 18/40)
USS	Pelvic – excluse twins and molar

Management

Acute	Admit, nil by mouth until stop vomiting
	Assess Hydration - skin turgor, mucous, pulse, urine output
Severe dehydration	Admit + IV Fluids (saline) + Electrolytes
	Folic acid + Pabrinex
	Thomboprophylaxis + LMW Heparin + TED stockings
	Anti-emetics (Promethazine, Metoclopramide, severe – Ondansetron)
	Weigh twice weekly until no ketones
Severe HG	Nutritional support (enteral or parenteral) may be required → if no response = coticosteroid

MISCARRIAGE

A miscarriage is the loss of a pregnancy during the first 23 weeks. 25% miscarry.

History

Pregnancy – HOW's

How many weeks are you so far? LMP? Was it regular?
How many pregnancies/children?
How was baby conceived? Planned or unplanned pregnancy? How do you feel about that?
How many scans have you had? (Must have had 2 scans - 10 and 20 weeks)

Miscarriage Specific

Bleeding	Colour, clotting, amount
Pain	Colicky, shoulder tip pain (ectopic), SOCRATES
Risk factors	Infections, trauma, age, alcohol, smoking, drugs
PMH	DM, connective tissue disease, uterine abnormalities

Patient care – WHO's

Who's at home with you? Any other support? How is everything at home?
Who is in charge of your care? (midwife/consultant)

Overall – check patient's mood and mental health

Investigation

Examination	Cervical OS
	Open - inevitable, incomplete, septic.
	Closed - threatened, completed, missed, ectopic
Bloods	BHCG, FBC, Rhesus
Baby	Small - incomplete, complete, ectopic
	Foetal heart at 6weeks
	Missing - complete, missed, ectopic
	Present - inevitable, present for threatened
Refer	Early Pregnancy Assessment Unit
	USS - viability & retained fetal products → repeat if doubt
IF recurrent 3 or more Ix:	Antiphospholipid syndrome antibody screen → Give asprin & LMWH
	Karyotype both parents → Give donor or PGS of IVF
	Pelvic USS → Give IVF

Management

Admit   Suspected ectopic or heavy bleed:
                  USS   If non-viable use IM Ergometrine (decreases bleeding)
                  Fever   Take swabs & IV antibiotics

Expectant   Wait 2-6 weeks
Medical   Misoprostol (prostaglandin) +/- mifepristone (anti progesterone)
Surgical   ERCP under anaesthetic

IF Rh negative & >12 weeks OR medical/surgical: **Give anti-D**

PRE-ECLAMPSIA

Incidence 5% pregnancies

History

Pregnancy – HOW's

How many weeks are you so far? LMP? Was it regular?

How many pregnancies/children?

How was baby conceived? Planned or unplanned pregnancy? How do you feel about that?

How many carrying - single or multiple pregnancies?

How many scans have you had? (Must have had 2 scans - 10 and 20 weeks)

Symptoms

Symptoms   Severe frontal headache?

Sudden swelling of face/hands/feet?

Abdo pain? (Liver tenderness/epigastric pain)

Vomiting?

Complications   Visual disturbance? (Blurring/flashing lights)

Any Bleeding? (HELLP)

> ### Specific Risk
> - First pregnancy/ new partner?
> - >10 years since last baby?
> - FHx pre eclampsia?
> - Underlying pre-existing HTN/renal disease/diabetes/APLS?

Patient care – WHO's

- Who's at home with you? Any other support? How is everything at home?
- Who is in charge of your care? (midwife/consultant)

Overall – check patient's mood and mental health

Investigation

Exam	BP, hyperreflexia
Urine	Urine dip, M/C/S
Blood	FBC, LFTs, renal function, U&E, Serum urate
Extra	24hr urine collection (>0.3g/24hr), clotting studies (< 100 * 10^6/l)

Management

MDT approach (obs team, anaesthetics, haematology, liaison with paediatrics)

Conservative   <34 weeks, haemodynamically stable, no HELLP

Refer if: BP >160 systolic or >100 diastolic
Raised BP w/ proteinuria => +1
Sx or signs of pre-eclampsia

Treatment:

If mild   6 hourly BP, don't deliver before 34 weeks

If moderate/severe   Oral labetalol is first line, nifedipine and hydralazine can also be used
AVOID ACEi (teratogenic, reduced fetal urine output), ARB diuretic

Prevention of seizures   MgS (N.B toxicity= Hyporeflexia, resp depression) + fluid restrict (max. 80ml/hr)

Delivery   Only cure- matter of balance between maternal risk and gestation
Only deliver if woman is stable

Prevention: Women at risk (HTN in previous pregnancy, CKD, AI e.g. SLE, APLS, diabetes) given aspirin 75mg OD from 12 weeks till birth

---

Classification of Pre-Eclampsia

Mild   Proteinuria + mild/mod HTN
Mod   Proteinuria + severe HTN + no Cx
Severe Proteinuria + HTN <34 <u>or</u> maternal Cx

POST-PARTUM HAEMORRHAGE

Causes

Infection - Endometritis (commonest)

Endometritis Risk Factors:

Caesarean section, prolonged rupture of membranes, severe meconium staining in liquor, long labour with multiple examinations, manual removal of placenta, mother's age at extremes of the reproductive span, low socio-economic status, maternal anaemia, prolonged surgery, internal fetal monitoring and general anaesthetic.

Retained products of conception (RPOC)

History

Intrapartum
How long were you in labour for? Was it prolonged?
Delivery: SVD, Instrumental or C/S
Any difficulties in delivering the placenta?

Symptoms
Have you had a fever?
Do you have any pain? Abdominal pain?
Have you had any vaginal discharge (smell?)/bleeding
Postpartum: Pain during intercourse? Pain on passing urine? FLAWS

Examination

General obs: Fever, Rigors, Tachycardia, Tenderness of the suprapubic area & adnexae

Elevated fundus which feels boggy in RPOC. Uterus is tender and OS is commonly open on speculum examination +/- remove placental fragments

Investigation

- FBC. Blood cultures. Check MSU. High vaginal swab; also gonorrhoea/chlamydia.
- USS - may be used if RPOC are suspected, although there may be difficulty distinguishing between clot and products. RPOC are unlikely if a normal endometrial stripe is seen. Ultrasound is not helpful in endometritis.

Management

For endometritis:

- IV antibiotics if there are signs of severe sepsis.
- If less systemically unwell → oral treatment may be sufficient. Antibiotic choice should be guided by type and likely source of infection
- The RCOG guideline for sepsis following pregnancy recommends IV Piperacillin/Tazobactim.
- For severe sepsis → Carbapenem plus clindamycin.
- For less severe infections → include Co-amoxiclav, metronidazole and gentamicin. However, guidelines based on **local resistance** should be followed

If Retained Product of Conception are suspected:

- Elective curettage with antibiotic cover may be required.
- Surgical measures should be undertaken if there is excessive or continuing bleeding, irrespective of ultrasound findings.
-

The patient may require iron supplementation if Hb has fallen.

90% of cases of postpartum endometritis treated with antibiotics improve within 48-72 hours.If due to RPOC, bleeding will characteristically slow down but will not stop. It gets worse again once Abx course is finished.

SMALL FOR GESTATIONAL AGE

Foetus below the 10ᵗʰ centile

History

Pregnancy – HOW's

How many weeks are you so far? LMP? Was it regular?
How many pregnancies/children? What was the previous weight (maybe it's normal)?
How was baby conceived? Planned or unplanned pregnancy? How do you feel about that?
How many carrying - single or multiple pregnancies (risk factor)?
How many scans have you had? (Must have had 2 scans - 10 and 20 weeks)

Complications – WHAT's

What was your booking bloods results – BP, bloods, diabetes?
What complications mum – blurred vision (HTN), pain, headache, blood loss? Tired (anemia)?
What complications for baby – feeling movement? Growth?

Patient care – WHO's

Who's at home with you? Any other support? How is everything at home?
Who is in charge of your care? (Midwife/consultant)

Risk Factors:

Smoking
Alcohol
Drug/substance abuse

Overall – check patient's mood and mental health

Management

Antenatal

USS	Chromosomal defects. Karyotyping may be offered
Screen infections	CMV, toxoplasmosis, syphilis.
Umbilical Artery Doppler	Absent/reversed end diastolic flow (pre-eclampsia)
If <36 weeks	Give steroids + deliver in a unit with neonatal facilities

Intrapartum

Continuous electronic fetal monitoring

Postpartum

Neonatal unit care   Monitor temp, give and monitor O2

Infection control (avoid crowding, wash hands)

Aim to breastfeed

Consider cranial ultrasound to detect haemorrhage.

Complications of SGA
Stillbirth
Intrapartum hypoxia
Neonatal Cx   Hypoglycaemia,
Hypercoagulability
Necrotic enterocolitis
Direct hyperbilirubinaemia
Impaired neurodevelopment
Later in life associated with obesity, CVD, metabolic Symptoms & T2DM

VZV IN PREGNANCY

History

Pregnancy – HOW's
How many weeks are you so far? LMP? Was it regular?
How many pregnancies/children?
How was baby conceived? Planned or unplanned pregnancy? How do you feel?
How many scans have you had? (Must have had 2 scans - 10 and 20 weeks)

Symptoms
Fever, headache, malaise, abdominal pain,
Itchy rash (head/neck/trunk, sparse on limbs)
Crusting?
Redness (superimposed bacterial infection)
Resp Sx of pneumonia (cough/SOB/sputum/chest pain)

VZV Specific
VZV	Ever had chickenpox/shingles before pregnancy?
Infection	Children well? Been in contact with anyone with chickenpox?
Vaccine	Had VZV vaccine? (Not routine)

Patient care – WHO's
Who's at home with you? Any other support? How is everything at home?
Who is in charge of your care? (Midwife/consultant)

Overall – check patient's mood and mental health

Information

< 28 weeks	Congenital varicella syndrome (IUGR, microcephaly, limb hypoplasia, chorioretinitis)
28-36 weeks	Shingles (dermatomal distribution rash) in first few years of life
>36 weeks	Neonatal chickenpox infection (especially if birth within 7 days of rash) and premature delivery
	In contact with chickenpox? How long for? (>4hr significant)

Investigation

1. Physical Examination – General examination, BP
2. Varicella antibodies (IgG)
3. Swab + PCR of lesion

Management

If not immune   Give VZIG up to 10 days post exposure.
<24hr rash/infected   PO Acyclovir 7/7
Contact avoidance

GENERAL PAEDIATRIC HISTORY

History

Frequency + Duration

When was the child last well

Systems review

Respiratory	Cough, SOB
GI	Change in bowel habit, vomiting, abdo pain
Neuro	Headache, fits, rash, joint pain
Urine	Polydipsia, polyuria
FLAWS	Fever, appetite, weight changes, sweats

Social – (BINDS)

Birth	VD/CS? Complications? Red book? Mum well?
Immunisation	Up to date?
Nutrition	Diet and food intake? Breast feeding or bottle fed?
Type of food? Fussy?	
Development	Have you any concern about their growth and
development?	
Social	How is everything at home and school? How is school
attendance?	

Development

Gross	Sits unsupported (**9 months**) walk (**18 months**)
Vision and Fine Motor	Pincer grip (**12 months**), transfer objects between his
hands (**9months**)	
Hearing and Speech	Three or four words (**12 months**), any concerns about
his hearing?	
Social and Behaviour	Smile (**10 weeks**) spoon (**18 months**)

Investigation

1. Physical Examination – General examination, BMI
2. Investigations – Blood, urine dip

ABDOMINAL PAIN

History

Frequency + Duration

When was the child last well?

DIFFERENTIAL	
Most Common	**Less Common**
Mesenteric adenitis	Lower lobe pneumonia
Chronic constipation	Obstructive cause
Appendicitis	Intra-abdominal mass
UTI	Diabetic ketoacidosis
Somatisation	HSP
	Hepatitis A prodrome
	Sickle cell disease

Symptoms

Pain	SOCRATES, waking up at night? School/food associated?
Vomiting	Area (Appley's Law)? Timing (cough, food)? Amount? Frequency? Colour (yellow, blood)? Projectile?
Stool	Colour? Frequency? Amount? Smell? Constipation? Diarrhoea? Floating? Undigested (toddlers)? Soiling (overflow)? Meconium (CF)? Mucus (IBD)? Blood (IBD, NEC)?
Mass	Swelling glands? Location? Swelling in the tummy? Distension?
Urinary	Frequency, urgency, nocturia, dysuria
Cough	Productive? Pain? (Pneumonia)
Infective	Preceding illness? Anyone else ill at school or home? Travel?

Systems review

Respiratory	Cough, SOB
GI	Change in bowel habit, vomiting, abdo pain
Neuro	Headache, fits, rash, joint pain
Urine	Polydipsia, polyuria
FLAWS	Fever, appetite, weight changes, sweats

Social – (BINDS)

Birth	VD/CS? Complications? Red book?
Immunisation	Up to date?
Nutrition	Diet and food intake? Breast feeding or bottle fed? How much/often? Type of food? Fussy?
Development	Have you any concern about their growth and development?
Social	How is everything at home and school? How is school attendance?

Investigation

1. **Examination**   General examination (Guarding/Rovsing's), BMI, cap refill, HR, RR
2. **Investigations**   Blood test, USS (intussusception, pyloric stenosis), CXR (bilious), suction biopsy (Hirschsprung)
3. **Stool**   Only if blood, septicaemia suspicion, travel

Red Flag for Constipation
Ribbon stool
>24 hrs meconium at birth
Distension
Amber Flag for Constipation
Faltering growth

ASTHMA (EMERGENCY)

General Observations

General examination (signs of agitation/impaired consciousness)
Resp signs (use of accessory muscles, wheeze, poor respiratory effort)
HR, RR
SpO2
PEFR

Examination

Children between 2 and 5 years of age

Moderate attack	Severe attack	Life-threatening attack
SpO2 > 92% No clinical features of severe asthma	SpO2 < 92% Too breathless to talk or feed Heart rate **> 140/min** Respiratory rate > **40/min** Use of accessory neck muscles	SpO2 <92% **Silent chest** **Poor respiratory effort** Agitation Altered consciousness Cyanosis

Children greater than 5 years of age

Attempt to measure **PEFR** in all children aged > 5 years.

Moderate attack	Severe attack	Life-threatening attack
SpO2 > 92% **PEFR > 50%** best or predicted No clinical features of severe asthma	SpO2 < 92% **PEFR 33-50%** best or predicted Can't complete sentences in one breath or too breathless to talk or feed Heart rate > 125/min Respiratory rate > 30/min Use of accessory neck muscles	SpO2 < 92% **PEFR < 33%** best or predicted Silent chest Poor respiratory effort Altered consciousness Cyanosis

Asthma Advice

Advise influenza immunisation every autumn

Inhaler Technique

1. Remove cap and shake
2. Breathe out gently
3. Put mouthpiece in mouth and as you begin to breathe in, which should be slow and deep, press canister down and continue to inhale steadily and deeply
4. Hold breath for 10 seconds, or as long as is comfortable
5. For a second dose wait for approximately 30 seconds before repeating steps 1-4.

To take a peak flow reading

1. Put the marker to zero.
2. Take a deep breath.
3. Seal your lips around the mouthpiece.
4. Blow as hard and as fast as you can into the device.
5. Note the reading.
6. Repeat three times.

COUGH

History

Frequency + Duration + Fever?

When was the child last well?

DIFFERENTIAL	
Most Common	**Less Common**
Bronchiolitis	Suppurative lung disease
Asthma	Inhaled foreign body
URTI	Heart failure
LRTI	Habit cough
Croup	Pneumonia

Symptoms

Onset	When did it start? Did it come on suddenly (foreign body/epiglottis)?
Sputum	Amount (XS = bronchiectasis)? Colour? Bloody (foreign body/TB)?
Nature	What does it sound like (barking = croup, whooping = pertussis)? Does anything come out? Bouts/fits (pertussis)? **Wheeze**
Timing	Recurrence (Cystic Fibrosis – infections)? Persistent/on waking (Cystic Fibrosis)? Night (asthma)? Better with night (habit cough)? Eating/vomiting (aspiration/GORD)?
Asthma	Night symptoms? School absence? Exercise tolerance? **Atopy** Eczema, hayfever (asthma)?
Other	Vomiting (pertussis)? Drooling (bacterial tracheitis, epiglottitis)? FTT (Cystic Fibrosis)? Coryza (pertussis, bronchiolitis, croup)? Chest tight (asthma)?

Asthma – (THIN CAP)

Exercise **tolerance**? Sports?
Have you been **hospitalised**? **Intubated**?
Night symptoms? Cough?
Control with inhalers?
School **absence**?
Smoking **parents**?

RED FLAGS
Blood in sputum
Sudden onset
Night sweats
Weight loss
FTT
RR > 60

Triggers – (CATPOLES)

Cold
Allergies
Travel
Pets
Occupation (near factory)
Laughter
Exercise
Smoking (parental)

Systems review

Respiratory	Cough, SOB
GI	Change in bowel habit, vomiting, abdo pain
Neuro	Headache, fits, rash, joint pain
Urine	Polydipsia, polyuria
FLAWS	Fever, appetite, weight changes, sweats

Social – (BINDS)

Birth	VD/CS? Complications? Red book?
Immunisation	Up to date?
Nutrition	Diet and food intake? Breast feeding or bottle fed? How much/often? Type of food? Fussy?
Development	Have you any concern about their growth and development?
Social	How is everything at home and school? How is school attendance?

Investigation

1. **Examination**   General + respiratory (Harrison's sulcus) + resp distress + throat swabs + PEFR + spirometry (<5, less coordinated) + sweat test (CF)
2. **Blood**   Raised WCC **or** eosinophil in asthma
3. **CXR**   LRTI, right lower lobe (inhaled foreign body)

Management

See Asthma section for Asthma management.

DIABETIC KETOACIDOSIS (EMERGENCY)

History

Can present with: Lethargic (no play), infections, drowsy,
                      vomiting, diarrhoea, collapse
DM Symptoms   Enuresis, polyuria (car journey), polydipsia,
                      weight loss, abdo pain, thirst

Have you ever felt this way before?
How controlled is their diabetes?

Systems review
Social - BINDS
Development

Investigation

- **Examination**
    - o Signs of gross dehydration (dry mucous membranes, sunken eyes, prolonged cap refill, decreased skin turgor etc.)
    - o Fruity ketones smell from breath
    - o Kussmaul's respiration
    - o GCS - Drowsy/impaired consciousness
- **Urine dip**
- **Blood** sugar, ABG, 12 lead ECG

Management

Immediate
If severe (hypokalaemia/GCS <12/SAO2 <92%/shock etc.) admit to HDU
Fluids Rhesus w/ normal saline; need to assess initial level of dehydration:
    If moderate 50ml/kg ORS;
    If severe, insert CVC, 20ml/kg bolus of 0.9% saline IV
    Mannitol (if signs of cerebral oedema: headache, irritability, red consciousness, slowing heart rate)
    NG tube is passed for acute gastric dilatation if vomiting or depressed consciousness

Insulin   0.05-0.1 U/kg per hr started after 1 hr

Aim for gradual reduction of about 2mmol/hr
Change to 4% dextrose/0.18% saline after 24hr when blood glucose down to <14mmol/L

Potassium   20mmol KCL

Acidosis   Bicarbonate

Re-establish oral fluids, subcutaneous insulin and diet

Long Term

MDT involvement (Community team diabetic nurse, GP, Dietician etc.)
Teach parent to give injection – need to take it forever
Teach parent and child about monitoring

Complications of DKA

- Cerebral oedema
- gastric stasis
- thromboembolism
- ARDS
- ARF

FEVER

History

Frequency + Duration
Previous episode?
When was the child last well?

DIFFERENTIAL	
Most Common	**Less Common**
URTI	Kawasaki
Otitis media	HIV
Pharyngitis	TB
UTI	Meningitis
Gastroenteritis	

Symptoms

Temperature	What is it? How did you measure it? Did it change?
Convulsion	Have you had one? What happened?
Other	Is he pulling on his ear?

Systems review

Respiratory	Cough, **SOB**, runny nose
GI	Change in bowel habit (**diarrhoea**), **vomiting**, abdo pain
Neuro	**Headache**, fits, **rash**, joint pain
Urine	Polydipsia, polyuria
FLAWS	Fever, appetite, weight changes, sweats

Social – (BINDS)

Birth	VD/CS? Complications? Red book?
Immunisation	Up to date?
Nutrition	Diet and food intake? Breast feeding or bottle fed? Type of food? Fussy?
Development	Have you any concern about their growth and development?
Social	How is everything at home and school? How is school attendance?

Development – determine if global (>2) or isolated

Do you have any concerns about his development and motor milestones?
Particularly his hearing?

Gross	Sits unsupported (**9 months**) walk (**18 months**)
Vision and Fine Motor	Pincer grip (**12 months**), transfer objects between his hands (**9months**)
Hearing and Speech	Three or four words (**12 months**), any concerns about his hearing?
Social and Behaviour	Smile (**10 weeks**) spoon (**18 months**)

Investigation

1. **Examination**   General + Neuro + Kernig + BMI + basic obs + Vision
2. **Blood**   FBC, blood flim, TSH, LFT
3. **Urine**   MSU
4. **If over 38**   Septic
   screen if over 38

Management

Traffic Light – see section

```
Measuring Temperature in a
           Child

Temp dot in axilla <4 weeks +
Tympanic membrane >4 weeks
```

```
              Febrile Convulsion

      Simple                  Complex
     <15 mins                 > 15 mins
    Don't Recur       Recur within 24hrs/same illness
    Tonic Clonic              Partial/Focal
    < 1 year old      Incomplete recovery at 1 hr

    Simple           More common, better prognosis
    Complex          Less common, worse prognosis
```

FITS, FAINTS & FUNNY TURNS

History

What do you mean by fits/faints/funny turns/seizure?

Frequency + Duration + Previous episode?

When was the child last well?

DIFFERENTIAL	
Most Common	**Less Common**
Febrile convulsion	Meningitis/encephalitis
Vasovagal syncope	CNS injury – incl. hypoxia
Breath holding attacks	Metabolic – hypoglycaemia,
Idiopathic epilepsy	hypocalcaemia (rickets)
	Infantile spasms

Symptoms

Before	When in the day? Warning? Witness? Illness? Fever? Activity at the time? Upset/ breathholding? Trauma?
During	How long? LOC? Limb jerking? Stiff or floppy? Tongue biting? Urine and bowel incontinence? Frothing mouth? Change in colour? Trauma? Eye rolling?
After	How long did they take to wake up? Fast or slow recovery?

Vomiting after?

Systems review

Respiratory	Cough, SOB
GI	Change in bowel habit, vomiting, abdo pain
Neuro	Headache, fits, rash, joint pain
Urine	Polydipsia, polyuria
FLAWS	Fever, appetite, weight changes, sweats

Social – (BINDS)

Birth	VD/CS? Complications? Red book?
Immunisation	Up to date?
Nutrition	Diet and food intake? Breast feeding or bottle fed? Type of food? Fussy?
Development	Have you any concern about their growth and development?
Social	How is everything at home and school? How is school attendance?

Investigation

1. **Examination** General examination + BMI +basic obs + throat
   swab
2. **Blood** BR (conj+ unconj), FBC, blood flim, TSH, LFT
3. **Urine** MSU
4. **EEG + MRI** Only if **recurrent** and **focal**. Not for **generalised** (only
   MRI).

Management

Epilepsy Carbamazepine (partial)
Sodium Valproate (generalised)

GLOBAL DEVELOPMENTAL DELAY

History

Frequency + Duration
+ Previous episode?

When was the child
last well?

<table>
<tr><td colspan="2" align="center">DIFFERENTIAL</td></tr>
<tr><td>Most Common</td><td>Less Common</td></tr>
<tr><td>Environmental
understimulation /
neglect
Iron deficiency
Cerebral palsy</td><td>Congenital/
inherited conditions
Brain dysplasia</td></tr>
</table>

Development –
determine if global (>2) or isolated

Do you have any concerns about his development and motor milestones?
Particularly his hearing?

Gross	Sits unsupported (**9 months**) walk (**18 months**)
Vision and Fine Motor	Pincer grip (**12 months**), transfer objects between his hands (**9months**)
Hearing and Speech	Three or four words (**12 months**), any concerns about his hearing?
Social and Behaviour	Smile (**10 weeks**) spoon (**18 months**)

Gross Motor (Limit Months)		Hearing, Speech and Language (Limit Months)	
Head Control	4	Polysyllabic babble	7
Sit unsupported	9	Consonant babble	10
Stands	12	First word	12
Walks	18	6 words	18
		Join words	24
		3 word sentences	36

Symptoms

Regression	Did he ever have any of these skills? Has he lost any of them?
Prematurity	Must adjust up to 2 years of age
Jaundice	Ever been jaundiced (kernicterus)?
Other	Previous meningitis? Does he use one hand more than the other (CP)? Hand wringing (rettes)?

Mum History

Any problems in pregnancy (APH/HTN)?

Has mum been trying to get baby to walk?

Does the child understand you? Can you understand your child?

When did the parents walk?

Family history of muscle or neuro disorder? Deafness/language delay?

Social – (BINDS)

Birth	VD/CS? Complications? Full term? ND? Asphyxia (CP)? Red book?
Immunisation	Up to date?
Nutrition	Diet and food intake? Eating from day? Breast feeding or bottle fed? Type of food? Fussy?
Development	Have you any concern about their growth and development?
Social	How is everything at home and school? How is school attendance?

Systems review

Respiratory	Cough, SOB
GI	Change in bowel habit, vomiting, abdo pain
Neuro	Headache, fits, rash, joint pain
Urine	Polydipsia, polyuria
FLAWS	Fever, appetite, weight changes, sweats

Autism Screen

- Does your child have problems interacting with other children/people?
- Does he make eye contact?
- Do you find he is overly obsessed with a certain hobby/toy?

HEADACHE

History

What do you mean by headache?

Frequency + Duration + Previous episode?

When was the child last well?

DIFFERENTIAL	
Most Common	**Less Common**
Tension	Meningitis/encephalitis
Migraine	Sinusitis
Myopia / hypermetropia	Raised ICP
Post-ictal	

Symptoms

Headache	SOCRATES – bilateral/unilateral
Migraine	Warning, unilateral, abdo pain.
	Triggers = chocolate/cheese/red wine
Vision	Diplopia
Meningitis	Fever & vomiting, neck stiffness, photophobia, phonophobia
Raised ICP	Worse on lying down, altered personality, early morning, sleep problems, vomiting
Concentration	Watching TV/screen? Missing school?

Systems review

Respiratory	Cough, SOB
GI	Change in bowel habit, vomiting, abdo pain
Neuro	Headache, fits, rash, joint pain
Urine	Polydipsia, polyuria
FLAWS	Fever, appetite, weight changes, sweats

Social – (BINDS)

Birth	VD/CS? Complications? Full term? ND? Asphyxia (CP)? Red book?
Immunisation	Up to date?
Nutrition	Diet and food intake? Eating from day? Breast feeding or bottle fed? Type of food? Fussy?
Development	Have you any concern about their growth and development?

Social	How is everything at home and school? How is school attendance?

Investigation

1. **Examination**   Neruo + Kernig + BMI + Vision
2. **Blood**   FBC, blood film, TSH, LFT
3. **Urine**   MSU
4. **CT**

Management

Acute	Nasal Triptan + NSAID (Ibuprofen)/Paracetamol (Not Pizotifan = weight gain +) → Aspirin = Reyes
Prophylaxis	1st Line – Propanolol and Topiremate Consider NSAIDs +/- antiemetic (promethazine)

International Headache Society Criteria - Migraine

A   >= 5 attacks fulfilling features B to D

B   Headache attack lasting 4-72 hours

C   Headache has at least two of the following four features:
- bilateral or unilateral (frontal/temporal) location
- pulsating quality
- moderate to severe intensity
- aggravated by routine physical activity

D   At least one of the following accompanies headache:
- nausea and/or vomiting
- photophobia and phonophobia (may be inferred from behaviour)

JAUNDICE

Jaundice is a common and usually harmless condition in new-born babies that causes yellowing of the skin and the whites of the eyes. Can cause brain damage.

DIFFERENTIAL	
Most Common	**Less Common**
Physiological	Biliary atresia
Breast milk	Hypothroidism
jaundice	HDN
Sepsis	G6PD/PKD deficiency
Feeding	Hereditary
difficulties	spherocytosis

History

Frequency + Duration
When was the child last well?

Symptoms

Onset	When did it happen? At birth? <24hrs? Persistent? How yellow?
Bowel habit	White pale stool (biliary atresia)? Smelly? Floating? Colour? Urine colour
Hypothyroid	Umbilical hernia? Floppy? Heel Prick test?
Other	Bruising, weight loss? Maternal blood?

Do you have any idea what your blood group is?

Systems review

Respiratory	Cough, SOB
GI	Change in bowel habit, vomiting, abdo pain
Neuro	Headache, fits, rash, joint pain
Urine	Polydipsia, polyuria
FLAWS	Fever, appetite, weight changes, sweats

Social – (BINDS)

Birth	VD/CS? Complications? Full term? ND? Asphyxia (CP)? Red book?
Immunisation	Up to date?
Nutrition	Diet and food intake? Eating from day? Breast feeding or bottle fed? Type of food? Fussy?
Development	Have you any concern about their growth and development?

Social	How is everything at home and school? How is school attendance?

Investigation

1. **Examination** General examination, BMI, cap refill, HR, RR
2. **Blood** BR (conj + unconj), FBC + PCV, blood flim, TSH, LFT
3. **Urine** MC&S

Management

Treat underlying cause, then commence either of:

Phototherapy	*A special type of light shines on the skin, which alters the bilirubin into a form that can be more easily broken down by the liver*
Exchange Transfusion	*A type of blood transfusion where small amounts of your baby's blood are removed and replaced with blood from a matching donor*

Most babies respond well to treatment and can leave hospital after a few days.

Use **chart adjusted** for gestational age & do: DAT- HDN (Rh disease)
ABO incompatibility
Warm/cold AIHA

MENINGOCOCCAL SEPTICAEMIA (EMERGENCY)

Management

1. Antibiotics
- < 3 months: IV amoxicillin + IV cefotaxime
- > 3 months: IV cefotaxime

2. Steroids
- if > 1 month and *Haemophilus influenzae* then give dexamethasone

3. Fluids
- treat any shock, e.g. with colloid

4. Cerebral monitoring
- mechanical ventilation if respiratory impairment

5. Public health notification and antibiotic prophylaxis of contacts
- Rifampicin

Management in PCT

Management if suspected meningococcal septicaemia and primary care:
- give IM/IV Benzylpenicillin unless there is a history of anaphylaxis (do not give if this will delay hospital transfer)
- NICE recommend phoning 999

Advice

Most children make a good recovery if treated early enough

There are several complications that may occur after having meningitis. These include:

Hearing loss	This is the most common complication. It is common to have a hearing test after you have recovered from meningitis.
Learning problems	There is a small risk of your child developing problems with their learning and behaviour.
Epilepsy	A small proportion of children have brain injury after meningitis, which can lead to epilepsy.

Kidney problems   A small number of children have kidney problems if their kidneys are affected as part of the septicaemia.

Joint/bone problems The septicaemia can cause some damage to different tissues in the body. This can lead to scarring to the legs, arms and body. Some people experience joint or bone problems which may develop several years after having meningitis.

MMR VACCINE

What is the MMR?

The MMR is a vaccine which contains weakened versions of live measles, mumps rubella viruses.
Why and when is it given?
It is given to a child soon after their first birthday when they are most at risk of getting infected by the viruses (because natural immunity fades from maternal antibodies).
The vaccine helps protect your child from experiencing the full blown symptoms of the viruses, if any at all.
The vaccine is very effective and is recommended as part of the UK Immunisation Schedule.

What is Measles?

Measles is a very infectious virus, spread by coughing and sneezing
Nearly everyone who catches it will have a high fever, a rash and be unwell.
Can have some serious complications:
- Chest infection
- Swelling of the brain
- Brain damage

What is Mumps?

Caused by a virus which causes a fever, headache and painful swollen glands of the face, neck and jaw.
Spread same was as measles and is about as infectious as flu. Serious complications:
- Deafness
- Viral meningitis
- Infertility
- Swelling of the brain

What is Rubella?

Also known as German measles spread in the same way as the other two viruses. This causes less severe symptoms and may even go unnoticed.

However, Rubella can be very serious for unborn babies of pregnant mothers. Serious damage to: - Sight
- Hearing
- Heart
- Brain

What are the side effects?

As with any medical intervention there are some side effects
The most common occurs in about 1 in 10 children who may experience a bit of a fever
There is a very small risk of about 1 in 1000 children who may have a fit caused by a fever, which is called a 'febrile convulsion'. However, to put this into context, if a child has not been immunised and gets measles they are five times more likely to get a fit (1 in 200).

Link with Autism

There has been some speculation in 1998 that the MMR was associated with Autism and that subsequently received quite a bit of publicity.
However, since then there have been numerous scientific papers written which show absolutely no risk associated
The WHO have categorically stated there is no risk.
The MMR is given at the same sort of time as the symptoms of autism appear
The doctor who published the paper Dr Andrew Wakefield has subsequently, been struck off the medical register. Dr Wakefield had shares in a pharmaceutical company that was trying to market an alternative MMR vaccine. The papers have also subsequently been retracted.

NON-ACCIDENTAL INJURY

History

Establish who has parental responsibility
Frequency + Duration + Previous episode?
When was the child last well?

Symptoms

Story	What happened?
	How did it happen? – Does the story make sense?
	Who was with her at the time?
	Time of presentation? – Any delay?
Associated	Does she seem to bruise easily? When did she acquire the bruises? Any pattern to the bruises - with a baby sitter or family member with her at the time?

Development – determine if global (>2) or isolated

Do you have any concerns about his development and motor milestones?
Particularly his hearing?

Gross	Sits unsupported (**9 months**) walk (**18 months**)
Vision and Fine Motor	Pincer grip (**12 months**), transfer objects between his hands (**9months**)
Hearing and Speech	Three or four words (**12 months**), any concerns about his hearing?
Social and Behaviour	Smile (**10 weeks**) spoon (**18 months**)

Systems review – look for chronic infections

Respiratory	Cough, SOB
GI	Change in bowel habit, vomiting, abdo pain
Neuro	Headache, fits, rash, joint pain
Urine	Polydipsia, polyuria
FLAWS	Fever, appetite, weight changes, sweats

Social (**BINDS** + Below)

Other children at home? – Safeguarding?
Known to social services?

Investigation

1. **Examination** General observations (look for withdrawn features), Skin laxity (Ehlers Danlos)
   Examine injury site
   Examine eyes (anemia, copper deficiency), blue sclera (osteogenesis imperfect), retinal haemorrhages (shaking baby)
   Inside mouth – poor dentition (neglect), torn frenulum (abuse)
   Skin – well demarcated lesions
   Red book and growth chart – FTT
2. **Blood** FBC (anemia + plt), CRP/U&E (infectious) + bone profile (Ca and Ph), clotting, X-ray (AP and lateral), skeletal survey
3. **Urine** Urine dip
4. **Imaging** CT/MRI - Subdural Haemorrhage

Management

Contact on call social services and Child Protection team
Inform senior paediatrician
Deal with injury/fracture
Document everything in the notes
Liaise with social services – consider Child Protection Case Conference

OBESITY

<u>History</u>

Obesity History

General	Height (GH deficiency), weight
Thyroid	Cold, constipation, tired
Medication	Asthma, headache, bruising
Prader Willi	Small hands and feet, small gonads

Food History

Intake	Portion size? How much food? How often? Weight gain over how long? Eats by himself or given food?
Dietary history	Talk me through what you eat in an average day.
Food type	Snacks? School meals? Fast food, takeaways

Exercise

Quantify	What exercise? Amount?
When	Sports? PE? Activity outside school
Lifestyle	Sedentary lifestyle: TV and games consoles
Symptoms	Any pain or shortness of breath?

Extra

Paeds Hx	GDM, IUGR, Child Red book
FH	Health of other family members

Systems review

Respiratory	Cough, SOB
GI	Change in bowel habit, vomiting, abdo pain
Neuro	Headache, fits, rash, joint pain
Urine	Polydipsia, polyuria
FLAWS	Fever, appetite, weight changes, sweats

Support (**BINDS** + Below)

How is everything at home?
How is everything at school? How is school attendance?
How does it make you feel?
Do you have friends?

Investigation

1. Physical Examination – General examination, BMI
2. Investigations – BP, TSH, glucose (GH), cortisol, clotting studies

UK 1990 BMI Chart	
91%	Overweight
98%	Obese
99.6%	Severely Obese

RASH

Frequency +
Duration + **Fever?**

When was the child
last well?

DIFFERENTIAL	
Position	**Condition**
Behind ears	Eczema, Psoriasis, Fungal
Flexors	Eczema
Shin	EN
Trunk	Viral Xanthems, Molloscum
Nails	Fungal
Mucous Membrane	Measles, Kawasaki, Herpes

Symptoms

Site (psoriasis)?	Where is it? Flexures (eczema)? Extensors
Onset	When does it come?
Character	Itchy (eczema, scabies)?
Radiation	Does it spread anywhere? Up to down (measles)? Everywhere (chickenpox)? Scarlet fever (spares face)?
Association	Systems review – esp. sore throat, URTI, fever, joint pain?
Timing	Does it come and go (urticarial)?
Exacerbation/Relieving	Allergens? Change in detergents/soap/medicine? Food? Sunlight? Pollen? Pets? House change?
Sepsis (meningococcal)	Fever, vomiting, headache, photophobia
FH	Atopy? Psoriasis? Asthma?

Systems review

Respiratory	Cough, SOB
GI	Change in bowel habit, vomiting, abdo pain
Neuro	Headache, fits, rash, joint pain
Urine	Polydipsia, polyuria
FLAWS	Fever, appetite, weight changes, sweats

Social – (BINDS)

Birth	VD/CS? Complications? Full term? ND? Asphyxia (CP)? Red book?
Immunisation	Up to date?

Nutrition	Diet and food intake? Eating from day? Breast feeding or bottle fed? Type of food? Fussy?
Development	Have you any concern about their growth and development?
Social	How is everything at home and school? How is school attendance?

Development – determine if global (>2) or isolated

Do you have any concerns about his development and motor milestones? Particularly his hearing?

Gross	Sits unsupported (**9 months**) walk (**18 months**)
Vision and Fine Motor	Pincer grip (**12 months**), transfer objects between his hands (**9months**)
Hearing and Speech	Three or four words (**12 months**), any concerns about his hearing?
Social and Behaviour	Smile (**10 weeks**) spoon (**18 months**)

Investigation

1. **Examination** General + Neuro + Kernig + BMI + basic obs + Vision
2. **Blood** FBC, blood film
3. **CT** Meningitis

Management

Treat the cause

SHORT STATURE

History

Frequency + Duration + **Fever**?
When was the child last well?

DIFFERENTIAL

Constitutional
Endocrine (GH/T4)
Nutrition
Steroid XS
Genetic/Familial
Infectious

Inorganic

Presence of parents/Neglect   Who is taking care of the child at home?
What is the height of the parents?
Insufficient food   How much food are they eating in a day?
Fussy?
Poor diet   What do they like to eat? Any special diet?

Organic

Swallowing difficulties
Absorptive problems   Stool floating? Smelly? (Coeliac, CF)
High calorific requirements   Chronic infection

Systems review

Respiratory	Cough, SOB
GI	Change in bowel habit, vomiting, abdo pain
Neuro	Headache, fits, rash, joint pain
Urine	Polydipsia, polyuria
FLAWS	Fever, appetite, weight changes, sweats

Social – (BINDS)

Birth	VD/CS? Complications? Full term? ND? Asphyxia (CP)? Red book?
Immunisation	Up to date?
Nutrition	Diet and food intake? Eating from day? Breast feeding or bottle fed? Type of food? Fussy?
Development	Have you any concern about their growth and development?
Social	How is everything at home and school? How is school attendance?

Development – determine if global (>2) or isolated

Do you have any concerns about his development and motor milestones? Particularly his hearing?

Gross	Sits unsupported (**9 months**) walk (**18 months**)
Vision and Fine Motor	Pincer grip (**12 months**), transfer objects between his hands (**9months**)
Hearing and Speech	Three or four words (**12 months**), any concerns about his hearing?
Social and Behaviour	Smile (**10 weeks**) spoon (**18 months**)

Investigation

Exam	Full examination
Blood (chronic)	FBC (anemia, infection) U&E (metabolic) TFT (T4) ESR/CRP
Urine	Urinalysis (nephrotic syndrome chronic causing short stature)
Genetic	Karyotyping (genetic)
Bone	Bone age

Management

Treat underlying cause

Give GH	GH deficiency, turners, Prader Willi, CKD, SGA

STATUS EPILEPTICUS (EMERGENCY)

Management

Immediate

Call Paediatric SpR

Secure airway

Apply facial oxygen and sat monitor

> N.B. if no immediate IV access, use **either** diazepam PR **or** buccal Midazolam (0.5mg/kg)

Check glucose and give IV 10% glucose 3-5ml/kg if hypoglycaemic.

Check temp and five antipyretic if fever

1. **Lorazepam IV 0.1mg/kg IV, to maximum 4g**

If no response or seizure recurs within 10 minutes then:

2. **Lorazepam IV 0.1mg/kg**

If no response or seizure recurs within 10 minutes then:

3. **Phenytoin 18mg/kg infusion over 20 minutes under ECG monitoring IV or if no access via IO**

CALL ANAESTHETISTS

If no response or seizure recurs within 10 minutes then:

4. **Rapid sequence induction using Thiopentone, intubation and ventilation, and transfer to PICU**

Advice

Outlook for epilepsy (explain outlook is better than many people realise):

- About 5 in 10 people with epilepsy will have no seizures at all over a five-year period. Many of these people will be taking medication to stop seizures.
- About 3 in 10 people with epilepsy will have some seizures in this five-year period but far fewer than if they had not taken medication.
- So, in total, with medication, about 8 in 10 people with epilepsy are well controlled with either no, or few, seizures.
- The remaining 2 in 10 people experience seizures, despite medication.

TRAFFIC LIGHT SYSTEM[1]

NICE traffic light system for identifying risk of serious illness in a child

	Green – low risk	Amber – intermediate risk	Red – high risk
Colour (of skin, lips or tongue)	• Normal colour	• Pallor reported by parent/carer	• Pale/mottled/ashen/blue
Activity	• Responds normally to social cues • Content/smiles • Stays awake or awakens quickly • Strong normal cry/not crying	• Not responding normally to social cues • No smile • Wakes only with prolonged stimulation • Decreased activity	• No response to social cues • Appears ill to a healthcare professional • Does not wake or if roused does not stay awake • Weak, high-pitched or continuous cry
Respiratory		• Nasal flaring • Tachypnoea: – RR >50 breaths/minute, age 6–12 months – RR >40 breaths/minute, age >12 months • Oxygen saturation ≤95% in air • Crackles in the chest	• Grunting • Tachypnoea: RR >60 breaths/minute • Moderate or severe chest indrawing
Circulation and hydration	• Normal skin and eyes • Moist mucous membranes	• Tachycardia: – >160 beats/minute, age <12 months – >150 beats/minute, age 12–24 months – >140 beats/minute, age 2–5 years • CRT ≥3 seconds • Dry mucous membranes • Poor feeding in infants • Reduced urine output	• Reduced skin turgor
Other	• None of the amber or red symptoms or signs	• Age 3–6 months, temperature ≥39°C • Fever for ≥5 days • Rigors • Swelling of a limb or joint • Non-weight bearing limb/not using an extremity	• Age <3 months, temperature ≥38°C • Non-blanching rash • Bulging fontanelle • Neck stiffness • Status epilepticus • Focal neurological signs • Focal seizures

[1] Nice.org.uk, (2015). *Traffic light system for identifying risk of serious illness*. [online] Available at: https://www.nice.org.uk/guidance/cg160/resources/cg160-feverish-illness-in-children-support-for-education-and-learning-educational-resource-traffic-light-table2 [Accessed 1 Jun. 2015].

URINARY PAEDS

History

Frequency + Duration + **Fever**?

When was the child last well?

Symptoms – (FUNDISH BD)

<u>F</u>requency	Of urination? Of drinking?
<u>U</u>rgency	Does he struggle to hold it in (eg stopping long car journeys?)
<u>N</u>octuria	Does he ever wet the bed?
<u>D</u>ysuria	Does he have pain when urinating?
<u>I</u>ncontinence	Daytime? Urine? Incontinence?
<u>S</u>uprapubic pain	Any pain?
<u>H</u>aematuria	Any red colour in your urine?
<u>B</u>owel	Have we got bowel?
<u>D</u>iet	Coffee? Carbonated fizzy drinks? When the **last drink** before bed is (should be 1 hour)?

> **Bed Wetting Questions?**
>
> Dry ever?
> Times in a week?
> More than once per night?
> Wake after wetting?
> Family history of bedwetting?

Systems review

Respiratory	Cough, SOB
GI	Change in bowel habit, vomiting, abdo pain
Neuro	Headache, fits, rash, joint pain
Urine	Polydipsia, polyuria
FLAWS	Fever, appetite, weight changes, sweats

Social – (BINDS)

Birth	VD/CS? Complications? Full term? ND? Asphyxia (CP)? Red book?
Immunisation	Up to date?
Nutrition	Diet and food intake? Eating from day? Breast feeding or bottle fed? Type of food? Fussy?
Development	Have you any concern about their growth and development?

Social	How is everything at home and school? How is school attendance?

Development – determine if global (>2) or isolated

Do you have any concerns about his development and motor milestones? Particularly his hearing?

Gross	Sits unsupported (**9 months**) walk (**18 months**)
Vision and Fine Motor his hands (**9months**)	Pincer grip (**12 months**), transfer objects between
Hearing and Speech about his hearing?	Three or four words (**12 months**), any concerns
Social and Behaviour	Smile (**10 weeks**) spoon (**18 months**)

"I understand it can be frustrating, how do you react to it? Do you ever discipline him?" (NICE says only positive reinforcement)

Information

Bed wetting – 10% of 5 year olds. 5% of 10 year olds. 1% of 18 year olds.

Causes	Very deep sleep, insufficient ADH

Management

Reassure. Treatment to above 5 only.

First	Rewards for agreed behaviour → not for dry nights. Don't drink before bed + go toilet
Second	Offer bell and pad alarm <7 year olds.
Short term relief	**Desmopressin** (esp. if travelling or bell and pad don't work)
Third	Refer to Paeds Specialist → Prescribe **Imipramine** or **Oxybutinin**

INDEX

Printed in Great Britain
by Amazon